Exercise & Health

A Layperson's Guide

By

Professor Kevin Sykes

A collection of short articles

Professor Kevin Sykes

PhD, MSc, Cert Ed, DASE, DPE, FHEA, FBAPT, CBiol, MIBiol

**Dean Emeritus International Development
Emeritus Professor of Occupational Health and Workplace
Fitness**

Professor Sykes has a PhD in Community Health from the Faculty of Medicine at the University of Liverpool and holds a personal chair as Emeritus Professor of Occupational Health and Workplace Fitness at the University of Chester. He has worked with surgeons, physicians and other health professionals researching the effects of physical activity and healthy nutrition on prevention and rehabilitation from chronic diseases. He is also author of the *Chester Step Test* and *Chester Treadmill Walk Test* – both used worldwide in clinical and workplace settings for medico-fitness assessments.

Professor Sykes has been a member of several Home Office Committees and Working Parties for the UK Police (ACPO), Fire (CFOA), Ambulance and Prison Services and has worked for many years with international fire brigades, police authorities and other corporate organisations to promote occupational health and wellbeing. He is a former member of the All-Party Parliamentary Group on Obesity, the Westminster Diet and Health Forum, a former Trustee of the National Obesity Forum, 2007 Scientific Chair of the British Association of Cardiac Rehabilitation and is a Fellow of the Royal Society of Medicine.

He is the author of 10 books, including a highly successful Penguin paperback, has published over 150 papers in scientific & professional journals and is a television and radio broadcaster, conference and public speaker.

Table of Contents

Take More Control of your Health

– become a regular exerciser

It's often said that we only really appreciate the things most dear to us when they're not there. This is especially true of our health, which most of us take for granted. Then, when we are ill, we visit our doctor and expect an instant cure by modern medicine.

In a recent public health survey, people were asked how much control they felt to have over their personal health. A large proportion answered 'very little'. These individuals also tended to rate their overall health status as 'fair' to 'poor'. However, those who rated their health as generally 'good', also reported feeling they had greater control and that lifestyle was an important factor influencing health and wellbeing.

It's an amazing fact that around 75% of illnesses in industrialised countries are caused by the *way we live*. Poor diets, lack of exercise and smoking are three major factors in seriously affecting our health and wellbeing.

Health is determined not only by the absence of disease but also by an individual's *resistance* to disease. But how do we make ourselves better able to resist disease.

The human body is amazing complex and regulates many of its functions within tight limits. This is termed 'homeostasis'. Whatever changes there may be in the external environment (e.g. a hot sauna, or a bitterly cold winter's day), the internal environment of our body cells has to remain stable. The body has literally hundreds of different control systems and the goal of virtually all of them is to ensure that the cells remain as constant as possible.

For example, if body temperature goes only a few degrees higher or lower than the normal of 37°C, this affects the life-supporting enzyme activity – which in turn affects our health. So, if we get too hot, our homeostatic control mechanisms are activated – and we sweat and/or go red in an attempt to lose the heat. If we get too cold, then we shiver and go white as blood is directed away from the skin to conserve heat. This is termed our 'stress response'.

If a stressor (e.g. heat, cold, and exercise) is applied often enough, the body will adapt. The summer sun of the Costas makes us feel hot, uncomfortable and sweaty when we first arrive, but after a week or so, we become acclimatised, we get used to the heat – we adapt. The first few days of a skiing holiday at 6,000ft can be exhausting because of the altitude, but after a week in the mountains, we've got used to it – we've adapted.

The early days of an exercise programme may leave you feeling stiff and tired – but after a few weeks it becomes easier and you can do more. Your body has adapted – you're now fitter.

Exercise can be considered as a real test of your body's homeostatic control systems – and the more vigorous the exercise, the more dramatic the test. For example, during a vigorous workout, oxygen is used up rapidly, lactic acid and CO_2 are produced in large quantities. Your body responds by increasing breathing, heart rate and muscle blood flow, mobilising energy stores and dissipating the heat generated by working muscles in order to prevent overheating. Activation of the nervous and hormonal systems helps to ensure that these responses are co-ordinated and efficient. After exercise your body then recovers back to resting levels.

Physical training results in a variety of changes to the shape and size of your body. There are changes in the functional capacities of your cardiovascular and respiratory systems. There are also changes in metabolic processes and cellular structures, such as an improved ability to mobilise energy reserves & protein resources and a more efficient activation of your immune system – all vitally important factors in improving resistance to pathogenic factors causing illness and disease. This is termed 'general adaptation'. Interestingly, these adaptations occur when you're resting or sleeping. That's why you need time to rest and recover. If your workouts are too heavy and too often, your body doesn't get chance to recover and adapt. So, the spiral is down and not up – and your health may suffer.

So, the effect of regular exercise is not merely limited to improving your fitness – your body actually learns the process of how to adapt – and applies it to a wide variety of other situations and stimuli, including resistance to disease.

If the exercise is regular and moderate, this adaptation process is very positive and highly beneficial to your health and wellbeing.

Looking and feeling good is a key selling point of regular exercise – and it helps make you feel more in control of your own health.

Health & Physical Activity

Would you be upset to hear that over 100,000 lives are lost, every year in the UK, for failure to apply a medically proven treatment? Well, it's true - our high-tech health care system has ignored a simple, low-cost therapy with the capacity to save hundreds of thousands of lives and millions of pounds. And what's more, we've known about it for thousands of years! The ancient Chinese knew about it. The ancient Greeks knew about it. In fact, Aristotle, in 300BC wrote that: 'a man falls into ill-health as a result of not taking it regularly.'! The Romans not only knew it - but their physicians actually *prescribed* it for health maintenance of their citizens more than 1500 years ago.

So, what *is* it.......this amazing wondercure?   Well, it's simply....**Physical Activity**!

The fact that regular exercise is beneficial for our health and well-being has been known for centuries.

Yet, despite us knowing this, a recent study from the USA states that as many as 250,000 lives are lost annually due to sedentary lifestyles.
Lack of physical activity is now considered as important a risk for heart disease as smoking, high blood pressure and high cholesterol. In fact, in developed nations, physical inactivity contributes to a over 30% of deaths from heart attacks.
This is made even more important by the fact that there are far more people who lead inactive lifestyles than there are those who smoke, or who suffer from high blood pressure or who have high cholesterol! Physical inactivity is a huge cause of premature death and disability.

Historically, we were an energetic nation of farmers, miners, labourers, merchants and travellers. An active life is one that almost everyone *had* to lead before we achieved industrial modernisation, technological development, the car, television, computers and labour-saving devices. Today we have the reputation of being an overweight, lazy, complacent nation, content to while away the hours with fast food, TV and video games.

The UK National Fitness Survey confirmed what many health and fitness professionals have known for years - that as a nation, we are not as fit nor as active as we should be. As a result of our sedentary lifestyles we suffer from a host of illnesses and diseases that affect our quality of life and shorten our *active* life span.

The Survey found that:

- Those who reported inactive, sedentary lifestyles generally showed poorer health records (even if they had been very active in their youth).
- There was a strong association between those reporting good or very good health status and those participating in regular physical activity.
- Those who reported participating in regular physical activity followed generally healthier lifestyles - fewer smokers, low alcohol consumption, healthier dietary habits - than those who were physically inactive.
- 7 out of 10 men and 8 out of 10 women were taking insufficient regular exercise to achieve a health benefit.
- Although 80% of the population surveyed believed themselves to be fit, one-third of men and two-thirds of women were unable to continue walking at a moderately brisk pace (3mph) up a slight gradient (1 in 20) without becoming breathless, found it very demanding and had to slow down or stop.
- Brisk walking on the level for several minutes constituted severe exertion for half the women over 55 years of age.
- Whilst activity levels decline sharply with increasing age, some elderly people were found to be as fit or fitter than others half their age.

An active lifestyle is therefore very important for our health and well-being.

But, how much is enough? And, does it have to hurt?

The answers seems relatively simple –

1. Aim for around 30 minutes of moderate physical activity every other day. This might include activities such as walking, gardening, cycling, swimming, dancing, organised keep fit classes and other recreational activities.

2. The idea of 'no pain, no gain, is really not true, unless you are involved in serious training for competitive sport. Try activities that will make you slightly breathless - like a brisk half-hour walk. You don't even have to get changed!

For those who currently don't take regular exercise, then begin with a few minutes of daily activity and gradually build up to 30 minutes. Try to build regular physical activity into your life and make it part of the way you live.
Add life to your years and years to your life.

'Walking is man's best medicine'
(Hippocrates 400BC)

For centuries we have known that walking is good for our health and wellbeing. The Victorians were famous for their 'constitutional' walks. Early evening promenades are still as common a feature of daily life in Mediterranean countries as they were generations ago.

Most people walk for pleasure - a family walk at the weekend, an evening walk with the dog, a lover's stroll, a hike or ramble in the countryside, walking around the golf course (the worse you play, the more exercise you get!).
In fact, UK surveys have regularly shown that walking is the most popular form of physical activity with British adults - way ahead of other sports and pastimes such as swimming, cycling, jogging, attending a gym or exercise classes.

So, what's so special about walking. Well, first and foremost, it's simple and it's natural. It uses your muscles for exactly what they were designed to do. It's controlled and rhythmical, covering the ground at a swinging pace that is fast enough to be rewarding, yet slow enough to be too exhaustive. You don't need to change into special gear, you can just step out of the door and walk. It's also a low-risk activity, where the likelihood of getting injured is very slight. So walking is a great activity for all of us.

People who walk for exercise usually enjoy walking for other reasons as well - they feel, in a vague sort of way, that it is good for them - not only in a physical sense but also in a mental and spiritual one. Walking does something for both the heart and mind!
Many people walk because it helps them to relax, to get away from the strains of living. A good walk can help iron out anger, frustration and tension.

At first glance, walking may not seem like much of an exercise to get you fit. After all, plenty of out-of-shape people walk. But in fact, walking can provide virtually the same cardiovascular benefits as distance running.
In one study conducted at our Laboratories at UCC, a group of sedentary 30-50 year olds walked briskly for 40 minutes, 3 times a week, for 3 months. On average, they improved their aerobic fitness

by 25%, their heart rates during exercise decreased by 10beats/min, they showed significant decreases in body fat and their lung function improved. They also reported feeling much better and much healthier - apart from the odd blister!

A classic study on London transport workers in the 1950s & 60s showed that bus drivers had around TWICE the incidence of heart attacks compared to the bus conductors. It was subsequently shown that a major factor in this was the amount of walking done by the bus conductors. The conductor on a double decker bus climbed the equivalent of going up - and coming down - the Empire State Building every day!

Another study from the 1980s on British postal workers showed that the delivery postmen had HALF the incidence of heart disease as the sedentary office workers. The walking element of the job was shown to have a significant protective effect.

Also, among those who take up exercise, walkers appear to have the lowest drop-out rates and report the fewest injuries, aches or pains. One study reported that the dropout rate from a walking programme was less than half that of most other activities.

Walking has often been called the perfect exercise because of its many advantages and astounding health benefits. Keep reading and you're sure to develop an urge to go for a walk......

Health Benefits of Walking:
- strengthens your heart
- reduces your risk of heart attacks and stroke
- improves your blood circulation
- improves your breathing and lung efficiency
- reduces blood fats and cholesterol
- helps weight loss and permanent weight control
- helps control blood pressure
- strengthens bones and helps prevent osteoporosis
- tones muscle and develops lean tissue
- reduces stress
- improves endocrine (hormone) functions
- improves self-esteem and body confidence
- improves your posture
- makes you look and feel younger
- gives you more energy

How to Start:
Most people don't require a medical check-up before embarking on a walking programme.
But, if you answer YES to any of the following questions, then see your GP for advice and medical clearance:

1. Has your doctor ever told you that you have heart trouble?
     Yes/No

2. Do you frequently have pains in your heart and/or your chest?
     Yes/No

3. Do you frequently feel dizzy or have spells of severe dizziness?
     Yes/No

4. Has a doctor ever told you that your blood pressure was too high?   Yes/No

5. Do you have any bone or joint condition such as arthritis,
that might be aggravated or made worse by exercise?
     Yes/No

6. Is there another physical reason (not mentioned) which might require
special attention in an exercise programme?
(e.g. asthma, bronchitis or insulin-dependent diabetes)
     Yes/No

7. Are you over 50 and not accustomed to moderately vigorous exercise?   Yes/No

Clothing & Shoes
Wear comfortable, casual clothes and a good pair of cushion-soled shoes, trainers or boots.
Dress for the weather and the terrain over which you plan to walk.

Walking Technique
- Try to walk tall with your head level and shoulders relaxed.
- Reach out your leg with your knee, heel and toe pointed forward in the direction of travel.

- Use smooth movements rolling from heel to toe.
- Let your arms swing naturally at your sides in rhythm with your stride.
- Breathe in and out naturally and rhythmically.
- Warm-up with some gentle limbering and stretching exercises.
- Cool-down at the end of your walk with some gentle limbering and stretching exercises.
- Begin slowly for a few minutes, then pick up the pace by quickening your steps and lengthening your stride.

Walking Tips
- "Walk and Talk". If you are getting breathless, slow down.
- "Listen to your body". If you feel pain, dizziness or nausea, then slow down and stop if necessary, to recover.
- Walk before a meal - or around one hour after eating, to give time for food to be digested (slightly longer if it is a heavy meal)
- Walk with a friend for pleasure and safety.
- Walk facing the traffic.
- Drink small amounts of water before, during and after exercise, particularly if the weather is hot and you are sweating heavily.
- Build up your fitness gradually over several weeks. Don't try to go too fast or too far, too soon.
- Try to make walking a part of your daily life.

Energy for Action

Sunlight - your body's energy source

When you bend your elbow, take a step or wink your eye, you use muscle power. But what exactly is muscle power and how does the muscle get its power?

It seems remarkable - but would you believe that your muscle power comes from *sunlight!* It's the same kind of power that charges the batteries of a space probe, or starts a fire when the sun's rays are focused through a magnifying glass. It is the radiant energy from the sun (which in turn is produced by the conversion of hydrogen atoms into helium atoms).

That solar energy gets into your body through the foods you eat. A process known as *photosynthesis* locks the energy from sunlight into the starches and sugars of plants. The sunlight is trapped by the green chlorophyll and used in the manufacture of **carbohydrates** from carbon dioxide and water.

These carbohydrates can be stored in your muscles and liver (in the form a substance called 'glycogen') to provide fuel for muscle power.

As your muscles use this locked energy, the carbohydrate molecule breaks down into its original components - carbon dioxide and water, which are removed from your body as waste products.

Your body can also get energy from its **fat** stores and, to a lesser extent, from *protein.*

 The fact that energy is released during physical activity is apparent as you feel your body heating up, causing you to sweat. In fact around 75% of all the energy released is in the form of heat, whilst approximately 25% is harnessed for muscle power.

Muscle Fibres - your body's 'action kit'

All of this chemical activity - molecules of sugar and fat breaking down to release energy to power your muscles - goes on in tiny muscles fibres, about the size of a human hair!

Your body has more than 600 muscles containing over *six billion muscle fibres* - varying in length from about one millimetre to several centimetres.

The smaller muscles of your eyes and hands contain fewer and smaller fibres than the larger muscles of your arms and legs.

Although muscle fibres are extremely small, they are capable of supporting over 1,000 times their own weight.

When groups of fibres act together, they can move your limbs in a powerful manner; the more fibres recruited, the stronger your actions.

Aerobic v Anaerobic

Food provides energy for action, just as fuel provides energy for a car engine. But the engine has only one way of converting fuel, whilst your body can shift from one energy system to another.

Anaerobic metabolism - instant energy

Your muscles can work for limited periods of time *without oxygen*. This is termed **'anaerobic'** work. During the few minutes of intense effort or lifting & carrying heavy objects, your body uses an energy store located within the fibres.

First, your muscles tap a substance called **ATP** (adenosine triphosphate). This is the only fuel that can power your muscles. But your store of ATP is tiny - and it burns out about one second. So, your body then uses another substance stored in your muscles, **CP** (creatine phosphate) to rebuild a fresh supply of ATP. This system supplies enough energy for around 10 seconds of intensive exertion. After that, your muscles begin to use a third energy source, glycogen (a form of carbohydrate stored in your muscles - with extra supplies stored in your liver) to rebuild the ATP. Unfortunately, this energy system also generates a substance called *'lactic acid'* - which builds up in your muscles causing pain and fatigue. When you stop exercising this lactic acid is flushed out of your muscles into the blood stream, enabling your muscles recover.

Lactic acid therefore, is the substance that causes your legs to ache - for example, when you've climbed a few flights of stairs.

Anaerobic energy is vital to us and it provides the instant energy required for the first few seconds of intensive physical activity and for the first few minutes of muscle endurance work.

Aerobic metabolism - the key to stamina & endurance performance

15

For activity to last more than a few minutes, we have to get our energy from a much longer-lasting source. This is termed 'aerobic energy' and relies on oxygen being supplied to your muscles by your lungs, heart and blood circulation. This is why aerobic fitness ('aero' means *with oxygen*) is often called cardiorespiratory (heart-lung) fitness.

The oxygen you breathe in and transport to your muscles then combines with molecules of fat or carbohydrate to provides the energy for **aerobic exercise** - such as walking, cycling and swimming. Aerobic metabolism is around 16 times more efficient at generating energy than anaerobic metabolism. That's why after a few minutes of exercise you settle into your **'second wind'**. Your body has gradually changed from supplying your energy *anaerobically* during the first few minutes to a more efficient *aerobic* energy system as you continue to exercise.

Carbs or Fats

At rest your body is using a mixture of carbohydrates (glycogen) and fats to supply its energy needs. During anaerobic exercise, your body uses its glycogen stores to generate the bulk of its energy needs (along with CP).

When you exercise aerobically, at a fairly vigorously intensity of around 75-85% maximum heart rate, carbohydrate (glycogen) is your body's preferred fuel.

If you 'go for the burn' with very high intensity workouts, then your body *has* to use glycogen and has to work more anaerobically as you near exhaustion.

However, when you exercise at a moderate pace - such as a brisk walk - your body will prefer to use fat as the fuel to rebuild fresh supplies of ATP. This is why L-S-D ('long-slow-distance') activities, such as walking and cycling are excellent 'fat-burning activities'. However, it takes around 15 minutes for your fat metabolism to swing into action, so a half hour brisk walk is ideal to get your fat-burning enzymes moving!

Fibre Types and Colours

Are you a Fast-Twitch or a Slow-Twitch person?

All muscle fibres are connected by nerves to your brain and they respond to nerve impulses. A nerve impulse is rather like a tiny electrical current travelling at speeds of up to 100 metres a second.

Some of our fibres appear quite *white* in colour and are connected to your central nervous system by high-speed nerves. They are called *'fast-twitch fibres'* and provide speed and high power movements. A top class sprinter would have a very high proportion of fast twitch fibres.

Other fibres appear quite *red* and are connected by less-fast nerves to your brain. These fibres are termed *'slow-twitch fibres'* and are better suited to more prolonged, endurance work. A top level marathon runner may have muscles containing 80-90% of these red, fatigue-resistant, slow-twitch fibres.

Most of us have a good mix of red and white - and various shades of 'pink' in between. Some of us have a higher proportion of white fibres and are better at strength and power activities whilst others are 'red-fibre folks' and are better suited to stamina-type, endurance work. Different types of fitness programmes will train these different fibre types. We can train for strength & power or for endurance. Each aspect of fitness will be improved best by training which is specific to it. So strength training is quite different to stamina training.

We can see these different fibre types in the sprinters and endurance performers of the animal world. For example, a breast of chicken consists of white meat - chickens are adapted for short, fast movements. Most game birds, such as grouse & pheasant, have pale pinkish-brown pectoral (breast) muscles, as they are flying sprinters.

On the other hand, pigeons, ducks & migrating birds have much darker, redder pectoral muscles and are well adapted to flying hundreds of miles non-stop.

There are also many examples where the two types of fibres are present in one animal - as in fish. If a grilled trout is laid on its side and the skin carefully removed, a thin line of red muscle (brown after cooking) can be clearly seen, which contrasts to the paler colour of the bulk of the muscle. This red muscle is involved in normal swimming, whilst the white muscle only comes into operation for more violent & powerful movements of short duration, such as when leaping rapids or caught on an angler's hook.

World-Class Sprinters & Endurance Performers

- The **cheetah** is the fastest sprinter - it can accelerate to 45mph in 2 seconds and reaches 70mph at full speed!! Its muscles consist predominantly of white, fast-twitch fibres. However it has little stamina and can sustain such speed for only a relatively short chase.
- A **flea** can propel itself over 200 times its own body length in a single jump!! (compare this to a Carl Lewis Long Jump of just over 5 times his body length).
- The **monarch butterfly** flies over 2,000 miles at an average speed of 75 miles per day to reach its wintering site!!
- The **humming-bird** flies over 1,500 miles across the Gulf of Mexico in 24 hours!!

Humans - all-purpose beings!

Whilst there are some superlative performances from animals, insects, birds & fish, we humans are designed as wonderful all-purpose beings. Individuals of our species can sprint 100 metres in less than 10 seconds, run 26 miles in just over 2 hours, cover 5,000 miles in less than 107 days (Max Telford ran from Anchorage, Alaska to Halifax, Nova Scotia in 1977, a distance of 5,110 miles in 106 days 22 hours), fly for one mile with the aid of artificial wings and swim the English Channel (21 miles) in less than eight hours.

In addition, we can produce movements of great precision, such as playing musical instruments, writing & typing, or striking a moving ball - all of which require extraordinary co-ordination. No other species is capable of this versatility!

The human body has astonishing endurance capabilities. In the animal kingdom only camels have been found to surpass humans in terms of endurance capacity. Australian Aborigines can wear down and catch kangaroos. Mexican Indians run great distances through mountainous terrain to catch deer. Navajo Indians can catch longhorn antelope - one of the fastest animals on earth - simply by wearing it down over long distances. A top ultra-distance runner (male or female) will easily beat a horse over a 100-mile race!!

Postscript

Your body is capable of generating energy for action in remarkable and elegant ways. But remember, in order for your body to work efficiently, it must be kept in good shape with regular physical activity and healthy eating habits.

Why Does Exercise Make You Feel Good?

We all know that regular exercise is good for us. It strengthens our bones and muscles, keeps our heart and lungs in good condition, helps us to relax and sleep better, helps keep our weight in check and makes us less likely to get sick.

But, exercise does much more than simply get us into shape and help us look good - it also make us *feel good*. The old adage "healthy body, healthy mind" rings true.

But *why* does exercise have this remarkable effect on us?

Scientists are still trying to unravel the complexities – but in simple terms, it's due to a number of "feel good" chemical messengers (hormones) that are released by the brain when we exercise giving us the sensation of wellbeing. These are often termed our *'happy hormones'*!

Three important ones are endorphins, serotonin and dopamine.

Endorphins *– the 'exercise high' hormone*

Endorphins are a powerful hormone released in the brain during aerobic exercise. Endorphins not only give the feeling of euphoria and exhilaration but are a natural pain-killer - three times more potent than morphine! Endorphins also increase pain tolerance and help reduce stress, anxiety, tension anger, confusion and depression. They also improve appetite control and produce an overall feeling of calm, pleasure, and general well-being.

Blood levels of endorphins increase up to five times resting levels during moderately intense exercise lasting around 30 minutes or more. Also, after several months of regular exercise, the body develops an increased sensitivity to endorphins (a higher "high" from the same level of endorphins), and endorphins that are produced tend to stay in your blood for a longer period of time. This makes longer duration exercise easier (you're feeling less pain!) and it causes your exercise "high" to last for a longer period of time after exercise.

Serotonin – *the 'hormone of happiness'*

Serotonin is a key hormone controlling our general mood. It is also involved in regulation of our sleep patterns, appetite, behaviour, memory and learning, sexuality, anger and body temperature. Serotonin is naturally produced in the pineal gland which lies deep at the centre of the brain.

Serotonin levels can become too low because of emotional or physical pressures, poor diet, too much alcohol or caffeine, smoking and no exercise. Low levels of serotonin are often associated with depression, anxiety, apathy, fear, feelings of worthlessness, insomnia and fatigue.

Whilst good diet and healthy lifestyle in general will help to improve serotonin levels, the most effective way of raising it is with regular, moderately vigorous exercise.

Studies have shown that serotonin levels are increased with increased aerobic activity after around 20-30 minutes and the production of serotonin stays increased for some days after the activity.

Exercise is a great way to increase serotonin and help maintain that feeling of 'happiness' and *joie de vivre.*

Dopamine – *the 'pleasure' hormone*

Dopamine has many functions in the brain and is commonly associated with the feelings of pleasure and enjoyment, with motivation, reward and positive behaviour. Dopamine has an important role in muscle movement control and coordination. In fact, low levels of dopamine in certain parts of the brain have been strongly linked to Parkinson disease.

Dopamine also helps regulate the feelings of fullness when we eat, so that we eat until we're reasonably comfortable and don't overindulge. But interestingly, a US study indicated that obese individuals have fewer dopamine receptors in the brain resulting in obese people eating more to try to stimulate the dopamine "pleasure" circuits in their brains.

However, not only can exercise can a 30-minute bout of moderately vigorous increase dopamine release but studies show that exercise can help increase the number of dopamine receptors, which can help stop the desire to over-eat. This has led scientists to suggest obese people may be able to boost their dopamine response through exercise instead of eating.

A 30-minute bout of moderately vigorous exercise stimulates the release of dopamine.

So, that's why a regular 30-minute dose of exercise is a wonderful 'prescription' to make you feel good!

Why Exercise helps Weight Control

Everything you eat contains calories and everything you do uses calories, including breathing, sleeping, reading and digesting food. Controlling your body weight depends the balance between the number of calories you eat and use each day. When you eat more than you need to perform your daily activities, your body will store the extra calories and you gain weight. When you eat fewer calories than you use, your body uses the stored calories and you lose weight. When you eat the same number of calories as you use, your body weight stays the same.

Whether you are trying to lose weight or not, regular physical activity should be an integral part of your healthy lifestyle. In many ways, it doesn't really matter what type of exercise you perform (providing that it is within your physical capability) - sports, gym sessions, household chores or work-based activities – all will burn calories.

There are basically SIX good reasons for incorporating exercise in a weight loss plan:

1. *Calorie Expenditure* – a 30-min session of moderately intense aerobic exercise will burn around 300-400 calories. Even a brisk walk will burn around 200 calories. So exercising for just half an hour, every other day will help burn around an extra 1000 Calories a week. Since 1lb of fat contains 3,500 Calories then each month this type of exercise alone will help flight the flab!

2. *Increase in post-exercise metabolic rate* – the longer the duration or the more intense the exercise, the longer your metabolic rate remains elevated after you've stopped and the more calories you burn. For example, after the 30-minute aerobic session, you probably burn another 100-150 calories during recovery.

3. *No loss of muscle tissue* – the effect of a low-calorie diet without exercise is the loss of lean tissue, which is not good for your health and will result in a lowering of your metabolic rate. This is highly undesirable as it makes weight loss even harder!

23

One study from the USA studied the contribution made by exercise in preserving muscle. This 8-week study on mildly obese adults showed that both the 'diet only' and the 'diet + exercise' (walk-jog/30mins/3xweek') groups showed a similar total weight loss of around 9kg. However, the *composition* of the weight loss differed significantly. The 'diet + exercise' group lost virtually no lean muscle tissue, whilst the 'diet only' group lost on average around 3.5kgs of muscle. Also the 'diet + exercise' group lost far more fat (8.9kgs) than the 'diet only' group (5.5kgs). In other words, for the non-exercising subjects only around 60% of the total weight loss was fat loss compared to over 95% for the subjects who exercised.

The scientific explanation for this is that in response to regular exercise, the body produces more growth hormone, adrenaline and noradrenaline. These hormones activate an enzyme called 'lipase' which breaks down triglycerides (stored fat) into free fatty acids, which are then used as a fuel during aerobic exercise. Resistance exercises also stimulate the release of growth hormone, which can trigger protein synthesis and muscle growth. Hence exercise stimulates the fat burning processes and helps maintain healthy, well-toned muscles.

4. ***Become a fat- burner instead of a fat-storer*** – a low-calorie diet without exercise will encourage your body to go into 'fat-storing' mode. If the brain senses that energy intake is too low, it stimulates the production of enzymes that will facilitate the storage of food energy more efficiently. This means that if you come off the diet, your weight will rapidly increase and may overshoot where you were before you started the diet. Regular exercise will stimulate the mitochondria in your muscles to develop fat-burning enzymes, so that you become better at burning fat calories.

5. ***Exercise is a mild appetite suppressant*** – interestingly, rather than make you feel hungry, research shows that moderate aerobic exercise can actually make suppress your appetite – so a pre-lunch workout or walk can often be very helpful within your weight control plan.

6. ***As you get fitter, you will be capable of burning more exercise calories*** – if you're out-of-shape your tolerance to exercise will be low. For many, even a 30-minute brisk walk may

be too far and a 30-minute aerobics class would be at a very easy level. For the unfit, the ability to burn calories is therefore very limited and a brisk walk may be at only 2mph. However, as you get fitter, your pace will increase and a brisk walk will now be at 4mph resulting in far more calories being burned every minute at the same moderate intensity of effort. You will also be able to exercise for longer. So getting in good shape not only makes you feel better but also enable your body to burn more calories during your work-out.

So, exercise not only helps control your weight but gives you more energy to carry out your daily lifestyle with vigour and alertness.

Combine Diet and Exercise for Successful Weight Control

The US-based National Weight Control Registry (NWCR) was established in 1994 and is the largest investigation of long-term successful weight loss maintenance worldwide. Given the common belief that few individuals succeed at long-term weight loss, the NWCR was set up to identify and investigate the characteristics of individuals who have succeeded at long-term weight loss. The NWCR is tracking over 5,000 individuals who have lost significant amounts of weight and kept it off for long periods of time. In fact, the average weight loss of people on the Registry is 5 stones and the average maintenance time is five years.

The scientists then investigated all 5,000 to find out how they did it and which strategies were most effective.

Here are the seven reasons identified by the researchers – and you might be surprised how easy they are to incorporate into your own life:

1. **Combining diet AND exercise is your best bet**: Of the 5000 people on the NWCR database, only 1% slimmed down by simply increasing their exercise levels; 9% lost their weight through diet alone, but a massive 90% gained their results by combining DIET and EXERCISE.
2. **Get moving**: The researchers recommend that if you're looking to lose weight you should aim to get about an hour a day of medium intensity exercise (such as brisk walking). Interestingly, they showed that turning off the telly helped enormously - those who spent the most time watching the box struggled most to take regular exercise and lose weight.
3. **Reduce your energy intake**: As you'd probably expect, most of the people on the NWCR followed a low-calorie, low-fat diet. Also, most reported finding it easier to control their diet on a regular basis than take regular exercise – until it was ingrained into their daily lifestyle.

4. **Be consistent**: If you're one of those people who eats 'good' food all week, and then lashes out on the weekend, you might want to re-think your strategy. Those who followed a consistent eating plan all week long (and didn't slack off over the holidays either) were twice as likely to maintain their weight loss compared to those who dieted in fits and starts.

5. **Eat breakfast**: Not surprisingly, one of the characteristics of people on the NWCR is that they regularly eat breakfast - most commonly cereal and fruit. It's worth your while to follow their lead, since eating a breakfast like this helps to top up your fibre levels, which helps you feel full longer, and thus decreases the likelihood you'll succumb to a mid-morning snack.

6. **Weigh yourself regularly**: 75% of these long-term successful slimmers weighed themselves at least once a week. By regular weighing, they were able to notice small shifts in their weight and initiate corrective measures when necessary.

7. **Steer clear of fast food**: One of the characteristics of people on the NWCR is that they ate less than one fast food meal a week. So, if you're the type of person who is constantly eating on the run, now you've got even more reason to choose something light and tasty like sushi or a salad instead of that burger!

But - how is it best to incorporate exercise into our lifestyles? We eat - and often plan ahead - our daily meals – particularly if you have a family or partner. But for many of us, exercise planning is not so easy – and often becomes lower priority.

For some, having a structured exercise programme is not a problem This might include visits to the gym, attending aerobics classes, swimming, playing badminton, tennis or other sports. In other words we schedule these in the diary and normally take a bag of kit and a towel for such activities.

However, researchers have found that in a typical week, many of us can actually burn far more calories in everyday daily movements when compared to living a slothful, sedentary lifestyle and incorporating a weekly gym session.

These calories have now been termed *'NEAT'* (Non-Exercise Activity Thermogenesis).

From where I'm currently sitting in a coffee bar with my laptop, I see two young women sat chatting. One sits very still, barely moving. The other can't stop moving. She gets up and curves between the tightly squeezed tables, just to get a napkin and then gesticulates wildly as she talks. She was saying how she wears a pedometer to measure the number of steps she takes each day and was well above the 10,000 recommended. But – she went on – "I put it on my three-year-old daughter at home who just 'just never stops' - and did 5,000 steps in ONE HOUR! The first woman, of ample proportions, said that she used to be just like that as a beanpole youngster – until her teenage hormones kicked in!

We now know that spontaneous energy expended in everything we do on a daily basis - getting showered, dressed, doing hair and make-up, fidgeting, housework, cooking, cleaning the car, walking up and down stairs, even working at a PC, walking the dog, etc, etc can add volumes to our total daily calorie expenditure. It is not surprising that NEAT explains the vast majority of an individual's non-resting energy needs – far more than a weekly visit to the gym.

So, the key message is to combine diet and exercise for long-term weight management, and if you can't make the gym or exercise classes, remember the very **NEAT** lifestyle way of burning those extra calories.

Don't Resist Resistance Training

The common hype is that fat-burning and weight loss is all to do with moderately vigorous aerobic activities and that resistance training is really only for muscle building.

However, contrary to what many people think, resistance training is as important – perhaps even more important - to successful fat loss as aerobic exercise.

There are several reasons for this:
1. Muscle is your fat furnace – it's where fat is most effectively burned - and resistance training will increase your lean muscle tissue
2. Muscle burns more calories than fat - a pound of muscle burns around 50 calories a day while a pound of fat burns 5.
3. Muscle takes up less space than fat so helps you look slimmer and leaner.
4. Resistance training increases your metabolic rate – enabling you to burn more calories you'll burn all day long.
5. Resistance training helps stop the loss of muscle that occurs with ageing (known as *'sarcopenia'*).

A hundred years ago, human muscle provided almost 40% of the energy used by our workshops, factories and farms. Today that figure is less than 1%. A generation or two ago people had to retain their muscle strength and power not only to undertake jobs in the workplace, but also do the day-to-day jobs in and around the home. People didn't need to go to the gym – their lifestyle was sufficient to keep them fit and strong.

However, life in the 21st century is different. Labour-saving devices mean that for many of us, there is just not the need for our muscles to remain strong in order for us to survive. So in today's world, rather than keeping our muscles as we age, we start to lose muscle after the age of 30, making day to day tasks gradually harder to perform, slowing down metabolism and increasing the risk of weight gain. We have to make a concentrated effort to exercise in order to save our muscles from shrinking and wasting as we get older.

Inactive adults typically lose around half a pound of muscle per year (more in females) - that's almost half a stone every decade. So our fat-burning furnace gets smaller - there is less muscle to burn off the calories. If eating habits don't change, we store the excess calories as fat and put on weight. Since fat takes up more space than muscle, girths gradually increase – dress and trouser size get larger as the middle-aged body starts to spread! The hour glass figure of feminine youth often becomes a beer glass shape in middle age!

Losing muscle is therefore not a good thing – it makes flab-fighting much more difficult. Whilst, aerobic exercise is a great way to improve heart and lung fitness and certainly helps keep your muscles in good shape, resistance training is much more effective at building healthy, well-toned muscles.
Males generally combine both aerobic and resistance training during a typical workout. Women tend to spend most of their gym time on cardiovascular exercise and tend to be more reluctant to undertake resistance training for fear of getting bulky. However, women simply don't have the testosterone levels to build big muscles – they develop leaner and stronger muscle fibres – with less fat between each fibre (intramuscular fat) – improving muscle slenderness and tone.

Significant gains can be made with a 30-minute resistance training workout performed 2 -3 times per week. A recent study of overweight women found that a three-month basic strength-training programme resulted in the subjects gaining 2lbs of muscle but losing 5lbs of fat – and all reported feeling fitter, stronger and healthier!

These days most gyms are well equipped with a wide variety of resistance equipment – and good technical instructors to advise you. However, remember to start with a resistance that you can comfortably handle with 12-15 repetitions. Move around the equipment, exercising different muscle groups in a circuit of exercises that cover the whole body.
Don't get overly-stretched on any exercise and move between the different exercises smoothly. In this way you get a good calorie-workout as well as effective muscle strength and endurance conditioning – both helping fat loss.

Resistance training has all kinds of great effects on your body:
■ Increases your 24-hr metabolic rate
■ Makes you stronger and increase muscular endurance
■ Makes you lean and slim--muscle takes up less space than fat so, the more you have, the slimmer you are
■ Strengthens bones – especially important for women
■ Helps you avoid injuries
■ Helps improve posture
■ Helps improve confidence and self-esteem – and body image!

So, don't resist resistance training – use it in combination with aerobic activities as a more effective way to control your weight.

Exercise and Syndrome X

Whilst one major reason to exercise is to help lose weight, regular exercise has also been shown to help tackle the co-morbidities (illnesses) that often accompany obesity. This condition is sometimes referred to as Syndrome X – or metabolic syndrome.

Syndrome X is a cluster of disorders including obesity, high cholesterol, high blood pressure and high insulin levels. In combination, these disorders dramatically boost your chances of developing potentially life-threatening illnesses such as diabetes, heart disease or stroke.. And if you are obese and unfit - your likelihood of suffering from Syndrome X is high.

Medical scientists have researched this group of risk factors for years, and have called it many names – Metabolic Syndrome, Syndrome X, the 'Deadly Quartet' and 'Insulin Resistance Syndrome'. Recent studies support what many doctors have suspected all along — that this syndrome is common and it's becoming even more prevalent. In the US, as many as one in four adults have Syndrome X, an increase of over 60% over the last decade. Worryingly, the statistics for the UK show similar results.

However, the good news is that leading a healthy lifestyle and keeping in good shape will help prevent Syndrome X - and, for those who suffer from the condition, lifestyle changes may help prevent before the development of serious diseases that will likely follow if nothing is done about it.

Signs and symptoms

Having Syndrome X means you have several disorders of your metabolism at the same time, including:

- Abdominal obesity, measured as a waist circumference of greater than 35 inches for women and 40 inches for men
- High blood pressure (hypertension)
- High fasting blood sugar (glucose) level

- Abnormal cholesterol and blood fat (lipid) levels — high levels of triglycerides (blood fats) and/or high levels of low density lipoproteins (LDLs - "bad cholesterol") and/or low levels of high-density lipoprotein (HDL - "good" cholesterol)
- Resistance to insulin, a hormone that helps to regulate the amount of sugar in your body

Having one component of Syndrome X means you're more likely to have other components of the syndrome. And the more components you have, the greater are the risks to your health.
One US study showed that women with three factors of Syndrome X are nearly twice as likely to have a heart attack or stroke and more than three times more likely to develop heart disease than those with none. The same study showed that those with four or five factors of the syndrome have nearly four times the risk of heart attack or stroke and more than 24 times the risk of diabetes.

Causes

Medical scientists now believe that the major, underlying cause of Syndrome X is insulin resistance. Insulin is a hormone produced by the pancreas that helps regulate the amount of sugar in your body. Normally, your digestive system breaks down some of the food you eat into sugar (glucose). Then your body uses insulin to transport the glucose into your cells (e.g. muscles), where it's converted to energy to fuel your various body processes (e.g. physical activity).

If your body becomes resistant to the action of insulin, glucose has more difficulty entering the cells. Your body reacts by churning out more and more insulin in an effort to help glucose enter your cells. This extra insulin helps maintain normal glucose levels in your blood for a while, but eventually your pancreas is unable to overcome insulin resistance. As a result, glucose accumulates in your body, ultimately leading to type-2 diabetes. Type-2 diabetes is the most common form of diabetes. It formerly was called non-insulin dependent diabetes (NIDD) or adult-onset diabetes. However, since this type of diabetes is now also found in children, this latter term is no longer used.

Syndrome X occurs before this point. Glucose levels in your body are abnormally high — not high enough to be classified as diabetic, but high enough so that the excess insulin in your system puts you at risk for other health consequences. The levels of cholesterol and triglycerides — another blood fat — in your bloodstream may increase, causing damage to your coronary arteries. And excessively high insulin levels may interfere with your kidneys' ability to process salt, which can raise your blood pressure.

The cause of insulin resistance isn't well understood, but it probably involves a variety of genetic and environmental factors. Doctors believe that some people are genetically predisposed to insulin resistance, and the tendency may be partly inherited. But being *overweight and physically inactive* are major contributors.

Treatment aims

The primary goal of treatment for Syndrome X is to prevent the development of type 2 diabetes, heart attack and stroke. Usually, this can be accomplished with an aggressive regimen of self-care strategies focusing on diet and exercise.

A healthy diet and regular exercise have vitally important roles to play ensuring that your body doesn't become prone to Syndrome X.

Exercise and Cholesterol Control

Cholesterol is something we've all heard about. It's been given enormous publicity over the past few years. Too much is bad for us.... can cause our arteries to *'fur-up'*..... leading to heart disease.

All true ... but that's not quite the full picture.... and it's not all bad news!

Cholesterol, is in fact, *essential* to our health and wellbeing. Without it, our bodies couldn't function, we couldn't even stay alive! Cholesterol is a necessary component of every cell in our body. It's found in large amounts in brain and nerve tissue, it's a building block for various hormones, including our sex hormones, testosterone, oestrogen and progesterone - and it's used to make bile acids, which are a vital part of digestion. So, cholesterol is not all bad news. But, the problems come when we have to much of it floating around our bloodstream. Then, it really does become a major problem to the health of our hearts by 'clogging up' our arteries.

So, exactly what is cholesterol?
Cholesterol is a fatty substance that the body can either make in the liver, or we can take in from the food that we eat. Cholesterol and other fatty substances, such as triglycerides (fatty molecules formed in the liver from the fat you eat or from other internal sources), are insoluble in water. To imagine what this means, think of trying to clean a greasy pan without using washing-up liquid - the fat just congeals and floats to the surface. The body couldn't possibly cope with clumps of fat floating around, so cholesterol and triglycerides are dissolved within particles called *lipoproteins*, then carried to your tissues in the bloodstream. This is a very efficient system of getting these essential fatty substances to all the body cells that need it.

There are three major type of lipoprotein:

Very Low Density Lipoprotein (VLDL).
VLDLs transport mainly triglycerides from your liver to your body tissues. If you eat lot of saturated fats, then you are likely to have

lots of VLDLs floating around in your bloodstream. High triglycerides levels are known to be an important risk factor in heart disease.

Low Density Lipoprotein (LDL).
LDLs are the mainly transporter of cholesterol to your tissues. If your diet is high in cholesterol, your liver will manufacture more LDLs to handle it - and your LDLs will be high. So, LDLs are often termed "the baddies" - and high LDLs levels are a major risk factor in heart disease.

High Density Lipoprotein (HDL).
HDLs are the 'garbage collectors', picking up unused cholesterol in the blood, transporting it back to the liver for dismantling and converting into bile acids to help our digestive processes. Some of the cholesterol is then passed out in stools, thus providing us a major route for the excretion of unwanted cholesterol. This is why HDLs are often termed "the goodies"! A high level of HDLs is now thought to be very important for heart health.

When you have your cholesterol checked, you are normally given a single value, say between 4 and 6 (the units are in millimoles per litre of blood – mMol/L) and likely informed that an ideal value is around 5.2mm/l. This is a measure of your Total Cholesterol (TC). Basically, this is the total of your LDLs and HDLs. However, what this doesn't tell you is how much of this total is 'bad' LDL and how much is 'good' HDL. Current research now tells us that whilst high TC levels are not good for cardiovascular health, perhaps more importantly may be the need for *high HDLs* as a key preventor of heart disease. Many doctors are now consider the ratio of LDL/HDL or TC/HDL as better predictors of heart disease risk, than TC on its own.
Additionally, a low level of triglycerides (TGs) is also highly desirable for coronary prevention.

Most certainly, diet can certainly help control your blood lipids (fats) and that's one good reason why low fat, high fibre eating plans are now routinely recommended. But exercise also has a very important part to play in controlling both cholesterol and triglycerides.

Exercise will help raise your HDL profile.....

Many studies have now shown that regular aerobic exercise will considerably elevate your HDLs. In fact, most researchers consider exercise as a more powerful factor than diet in raising HDLs. Our own recent studies at University College Chester noted a 35% in HDLs with a group of sedentary ladies who undertook an 8-week course of moderately vigorous low impact aerobics. Women tend to have a naturally higher HDL level than men, so the potential for improving HDLs amongst males is significant. This is now thought to be one of the most significant reasons for the dramatic drop in coronary risk for active males.

Exercise will help lower your triglycerides.....
Significant changes in TGs have been shown by many researchers. One recent North American study reported a fall of 43% in TGs amongst a group of sedentary men and women who were asked to engage in aerobic exercise, such as brisk walking, for around 30 minutes, 3-4 times a week. Your body uses the TGs as a fuel for aerobic exercise - so exercise is a great way to lower your triglycerides.

Total Cholesterol and LDLs are also shown to be lower in active people, largely due to the generally healthier lifestyle, such as good eating habits, not smoking and moderate alcohol consumption.

Controlling blood fat levels is a key feature in improving the health of your heart.
A combination of low fat, high fibre healthy eating habits and taking regular aerobic physical activity are powerful ways of exercising this cholesterol control.

So, keep your blood profile healthy – eat sensibly and exercise regularly.

Exercise and the Common Cold

- a walk a day keeps the doctor at bay...

A cold is an inflammation of the upper respiratory tract caused by a viral infection. The common cold is probably the most frequently occurring illness in humans worldwide. More than 200 different viruses cause colds, and rhinoviruses and coronaviruses are the culprits 25-60 percent of the time. Rhinovirus infections often occur during the fall and spring seasons, while the coronavirus is more common during the winter.

The U.S. Centers for Disease Control and prevention estimates that over 425 million colds and bouts of flu occur annually in the united States, resulting in $2.5 billion in lost school and work days, and in medical costs. The average person has two or three respiratory infections per year. Young children suffer from six to seven annually.

How do you catch a cold?

Although still a matter of controversy, growing evidence suggests that at
least among adults, cold viruses are passed from person to person primarily
by being inhaled into the nose and air passageways (*i.e.* spread
through the air). Severe colds transmit viruses more readily than mild ones
because a greater amount of virus is passed into the air by coughing and
sneezing. Thus, to hinder the spread of cold viruses, coughs, sneezes
and "nose-blows" should be smothered with clean handkerchiefs or facial tissues. Contrary to popular opinion, damp, cold or drafty weather does *not* increase the risk of getting a cold. According to most cold researchers, cold or bad weather simply brings people together indoors, which leads to more person-to-person contact.

Cold Treatment

Doctors often quip that a cold lasts seven days without treatment, and one week with it! Most non-prescription medications, such as antihistamines, decongestants, cough medicines, and analgesics provide only temporary relief of symptoms. These medications can make you feel more comfortable while your body's immune system gears up to fight off the infection. To get rid of the cold, your immune system must make enough antibodies to destroy the viruses, a process that takes three to four days.

Antibiotics that fight bacteria have no value in the treatment of the uncomplicated common cold which is caused by a virus. Even the old standby - inhaling steam -- has little or no beneficial effect on cold symptoms! Vitamin C does not prevent colds, according to most researchers, but may slightly reduce the severity and duration of symptoms. Resting, drinking plenty of hot fluids, and seeking comfort from over-the-counter cold remedies is still all that can be done to treat most colds.

Keep your immune system in good shape

Whether you actually get sick from a cold after a sufficient amount of the virus has entered your body depends on many factors that affect your immune system. Smoking, stress, poor nutrition and lack of sleep have all been associated with impaired immune function and increased risk of infection.

So, your immune system can be strengthened – and your defences against disease fortified - by eating a well-balanced diet, keeping life stresses to a minimum, avoiding chronic fatigue and obtaining adequate sleep. For weight watchers, immune function is suppressed during periods of very low caloric intake and quick weight reduction, so weight loss should be gradual to maintain good immunity.

Can a walk each day keep the doctor at bay?

People who exercise report fewer colds than their inactive peers. For example, one recent survey revealed that 61% of 700 recreational runners reported fewer colds since beginning to run, while only 4 percent felt they experienced more. In another survey of 170 experienced runners who had been training for 12 years, 90% reported that they definitely or mostly agreed with the statement that they "rarely get sick."

To test this belief scientifically, two well-controlled studies with young and elderly women were conducted. In both studies, women in the exercise groups walked briskly 35-45 minutes, five days a week, for 12-15 weeks, with the control groups remained physically inactive. The results were in the same direction reported by fitness enthusiasts – the regular walkers experienced about half the days with cold symptoms as the sedentary controls.

Other research has shown that during moderate exercise, several positive changes occur in the immune system. Although the immune system returns to pre-exercise levels very quickly after the exercise session is over, each session represents a boost that appears to reduce the risk of infection over the long term.

A study in Hong Kong

Can too much exercise lower your resistances?

Among elite athletes and their coaches, a common perception is that heavy exertion reduces resistance to colds. During the 1998 Winter and Summer Olympic Games, team doctors reported that "upper respiratory infections abound" and that "the most irksome troubles with athletes are viral infections." To determine whether these anecdotal reports were true, 2,311 marathon runners who ran the recent Los Angeles Marathon were studied. During the week following the race, one out of seven runners became sick, which was about five times the rate of runners who trained for, but did not run, the Marathon. During the two-month period before the race, runners training more than 60 miles a week doubled their odds for sickness compared to those training less than 20 miles a week. Researchers in South Africa have also confirmed that after marathon-type exertion, runners are at a high risk for sickness. The immune systems of marathon runners have been studied under laboratory conditions before and after running 2-3 hours. A steep drop in immune function occurs lasting at least 6-9 hours. Several exercise immunologists believe this allows viruses to spread and gain a foothold. Overdoing your exercise can lower your resistance and adversely affect your ability to keep the colds at bay.

So, a walk a day really can help keep the doctor at bay!

The Exercise-Cancer Connection

Although heart disease is our number one killer, many of us fear cancer the most.

More than 100 different types of cancer exist. The leading cancer killer for both men and women is lung cancer, followed by breast, prostate and bowel (colon) cancer. In the US, cancer is now the leading cause of death in young women between the ages of 25 and 44 years. About 35% of cancers are attributed to dietary factors (e.g. high fat, low fibre) and around 30% due to smoking. The American Cancer Society recommends avoiding all tobacco use and eating a low-fat, high fibre diet containing plenty of wholegrains, fruits and vegetables in order to reduce cancer risk. However, evidence is now mounting that our sedentary lifestyles may contribute significantly to the development of cancer. So much so, that in 1996, the American Cancer Society added *physical activity* as an important preventive measure.

That exercise may provide some protection against cancer is not new. Studies conducted in the 1920s made these observations but it is only in the last decade that medical scientists have re-opened the casebook. Since then many studies have confirmed an exercise-cancer prevention connection.

One of the most common forms of cancer in white females over 40 is breast cancer and is the leading cause of death in women between the ages of 40 and 60. Main risk factors include family history, first menstrual period at an early age, menopause at a late age, first childbirth after 30, or no childbirth and a high-fat diet. Until relatively recently, many women assumed they had no control over preventing breast cancer if they had a strong predisposition to the disease.

However, a recent study by Leslie Bernstein, professor of preventive medicine at California's Norris Cancer Centre revealed statistics to the contrary. She found that women who had been habitually active from the time they started menstruating were 30-60% less likely to develop breast cancer by the age of 40, than non-exercisers. Furthermore, a study in Washington DC which reviewed the death records of 25,000 women, revealed that those who had worked in physically demanding jobs had significantly fewer deaths from breast cancer. Another US study on 16,000 women showed that

41

those who took regular aerobic exercise had a 50% reduction in breast cancer risk. Norwegian scientists investigating 26,000 women found that those who were regular exercisers had overall 37% fewer breast cancers than those who were sedentary – but interestingly showed that the risk of breast cancer was 72% lower in *lean* women who exercised regularly compared to the non-exercisers.

Exercise can also help to lower risk of developing other female reproductive cancers. Although research is limited, there is increasing evidence to show that regular exercisers are at significantly less risk for both ovarian and uterine cancers than sedentary women.

How does exercise help lower breast cancer risk?

Medical scientists have discovered that regular moderate exercise lowers the body's production of two ovarian hormones (oestradiol – a type of oestrogen - and progesterone) linked to breast tumour development. The body's susceptibility to oestradiol and progesterone is greatest between ovulation and the beginning of menstruation. Regular exercise appears to postpone ovulation until later in the woman's monthly cycle, thereby reducing the number of days her body must combat these potentially harmful hormones. In addition, regular moderate exercise burns fat, a pre-requisite for oestrogen production. So the fat which is used to manufacture unwanted amounts of oestrogen is used in fat-burning exercise.

It has also been found that in pre-pubescents, girls who exercise regularly tend to get their first periods up to several years later than sedentary girls and physically active young girls who have started menstruating may not actually ovulate until later. Reducing the number of ovulations that a woman experiences over a lifetime means less exposure to oestrogens and progesterone.

Leanness is also important, since as body fat levels increase so generally does the level of oestradiol. For this reason, many researchers feel that the reduction of body fat with regular exercise may be one of the key protective mechanisms against breast cancer.

Other exercise-cancer protection mechanisms

The fortification of the body's immune system that results from regular moderate physical activity is also thought to play a key role in lowering cancer risk. *Natural Killer (NK) cells* are an important part of the immune system and provide a first line of defence against various pathogens. They have the ability to inactivate viruses and have an anti-tumour action, helping prevent the metastatic growth potential of cancerous cells. Other immune system cells, known as *T-cells* also defend against viral and fungal infections, help destroy cancer cells and prevent tumour growth. Regular moderate exercise is known to boost the levels of both NK and T-cell activity and thus help the body defend itself against illness.

Regular exercise can also reduce levels of glucose and insulin and increase levels of corticosteroid hormones, which reduces cancer risk. Exercise increases interferon production and improves metabolism of ascorbic acid (Vitamin C) - which may both help prevent the formation cancerous tumours. Other potential effects of exercise in the prevention of cancer include beneficial changes to the body's antioxidant functions and prostaglandin metabolism.

The role of exercise in lowering colon and prostate cancer risk
Numerous investigations have shown that people who have sedentary lifestyles have significantly greater risk of developing colon cancer. Of 35 studies conducted worldwide, 30 showed that physically active people have significantly less colon cancer than sedentary counterparts. Research at Harvard University on over 48,000 health workers revealed that colon cancer risk was 50% lower in people who took regular exercise compared to those who led sedentary lifestyles. Another study showed that 2 hours a week or more of moderately vigorous physical activity lowered the risk of colon cancer by 40%. It seems that improved bowel movements (peristalsis), often seen in regular exercisers, shortens the time that various cancer-producing chemicals stay in the colon. It is well reported that regular exercisers suffer less from constipation than sedentary people. So exercise has an effect on the colon rather like that of dietary fibre. In addition, obesity and inactivity lead to higher blood insulin levels (a hormone that can affect the colon-lining cells). Regular exercise promotes leanness and reduces insulin levels.

There are only about 15 studies investigating physical activity and prostate cancer and findings are mixed. However, around half of them showed that physical inactivity was a significant risk factor. A 16-year study in Norway on 53,000 men found that the risk of prostate cancer was reduced by 50% in those over-60s who walked regularly during their work and leisure-time. Research in Dallas revealed a 74% reduction in developing prostate cancer when comparing 'low fitness-inactive' with 'high fitness-regularly active' groups of men.

Research has found that physically fit, active individuals have overall, around four times less cancer than their sedentary counterparts.
So, regular moderate exercise can play a significant role in reducing your cancer risk.
Good health, good fitness – stay active.

Footnote:

Exercise for cancer patients
Whilst it is generally thought that exercise does not help treat cancer once it is formed, many physicians now recommend regular exercise to cancer patients to improve fitness, life quality, self-esteem and morale.
However, the exercise should be symptom-limited, progressive and individualised. Providing there are no specific contraindications to exercise, general ambulation is generally encouraged for most sedentary and deconditioned cancer patients. Short bouts of exercise of around 5-10 minutes, including aerobic activities such as walking, coupled with exercises to improve range of joint motion, general flexibility and muscle strength are often prescribed. As the patient improves, this may be built up to more continuous exercise sessions lasting 15-20 minutes.
Whilst there is limited research on the role of exercise in cancer rehabilitation, the available data suggest a strong psychological role for regular physical activity.
One recent US study showed that breast cancer patients exercising for 30 minutes, 4 days a week showed significantly less depression scores and more self-esteem than non-exercising counterparts.
For most cancer sufferers, loss of body mass and 'functional fitness' are amongst the serious outcomes. The loss of 'functional fitness' includes difficulty in doing household jobs such as cleaning, vacuuming, washing & ironing, difficulty in walking and climbing stairs. Over 75% of cancer survivors report extreme feelings of fatigue during radiotherapy and chemotherapy, which are associated with loss of weight, loss of muscle, strength and cardiovascular endurance. Maintaining and restoring this 'functional fitness' are challenges for the cancer survivor - even those patients

who are considered 'cured'. Studies show that regular, moderate physical activity - a combination of aerobic and resistance exercises - can significantly assist recovery in cancer survivors. An increased level of activity will assist the patient to return to physical independence and an improving quality of life.

Exercise and SAD

.....Keep Away Those Winter Blues

These winter months have many of us reaching for the holiday brochures. Winter Sun is now huge business for the travel trade with millions of us searching for the sunshine at this time of year. Rain, wind, cloudy weather, cold and lack of sunshine are all normal features of a British winter that many of us find utterly depressing. In fact some of us show a very different pattern of behaviour when the seasons change. For example:

In winter:
1. Do you find you have less energy than in summer?
2. Do you find it harder to get out of bed in the morning?
3. Do you sleep more but still wake up feeling tired?
4. Do you feel more stressed?
5. Do you feel more depressed?
6. Do you put on weight?
7. Do you suffer more from pre-menstrual tension?
8. Do you find it more difficult to get enthusiastic about things?

If you answer 'Yes' to more than two of the above questions, you may be one of the many who are affected, to a greater or lesser extent, by a condition termed 'Seasonal Affective Disorder' (SAD). In the USA, it is estimated that over 35 million people suffer in one way or another from SAD - or 'winter blues'. What's interesting is that it doesn't appear to trouble people living in Florida and the Southern States as much as those living in New Hampshire and the northern Great Lakes States. And in Europe, it's a far bigger problem for those living in Norway and Sweden than for those in Mediterranean countries. The studies also show that women are around 3-4 times as likely to suffer from 'winter blues' as men. The problem seem to affect 20-40 year olds in particular, with reports of lethargy, fatigue, ravenous appetite, weight gain, carbohydrate craving, withdrawal from relationships, inability to concentrate or focus, problems at work, anxiety and despair during the winter months.

'Winter blues' or SAD is thought to be brought on by lack of daylight. In summer, the days are long and the light is generally bright. But in a British winter, the days are short and the light is generally of poor quality. It is only during the last decade or so that scientists have really begun to understand the importance of natural daylight to out health and vitality.

Daylight enters our eyes (even when our eyes are closed) and sends signals to the pineal gland, located at the centre of the brain. Bright light causes a whole series of physiological responses and changes in the body. The morning sun wakes us up, whereas at night-time the darkness stimulates production of the hormone melatonin, which makes us feel drowsy and sleepy. During long summer days, more endorphins and serotonin are produced in the brain - these are neurotransmitters which make us feel better, more energetic, less depressed and less moody.

Being outdoors in daylight also encourages the production of more Vitamin D, which is manufactured in the skin as a result of exposure to daylight. This promotes better absorption of calcium, phosphorus and magnesium, which strengthen our bones & teeth and are essential in combating arthritis, osteoporosis and the negative effects of the menopause. In spring, when the days begin to lengthen, our sex hormones take a surge forward. Indeed the peak time for conception is late spring and early summer. A young man's fancy....and all that!

The Ancient Greeks recognised the importance of daylight to health and fitness by training outdoors naked, thus exposing all of their muscles to gain a beneficial effect from the sunlight! The Victorians had their 'morning constitutional walk', whilst from the turn of the century up to the Second World War, sanatoriums were built to enable patients to sit outside and receive daily exposures to sunlight as a part of the treatment.

Interestingly, a recent report from the USA found that heart patients whose beds were on the sunny-side of the ward recovered faster than other patients! Was this just coincidence?

Some current experts are now suggesting that fitness training outdoors is more beneficial than an indoor workout. When the skin is exposed to daylight the capacity of the blood for transporting oxygen goes up, more oxygen and nutrients are supplied to the tissues and muscles become better toned. Some research also suggests that we are better able to fat-burn when we exercise outdoors in natural daylight. Several offices and gymnasia now have full-spectrum lighting and whilst there have been some problems, most report good effects.

Many of us lead lifestyles where as much as 90% of our time is spent indoors, away from natural daylight. We travel to work in a car, bus or train, work indoors, lunch indoors, return home and spend our leisure time indoors. Why is it that shift workers have more health problems than the rest of us? More stress, less exercise, more smokers - or could it be light-deficiency?

Curing or keeping away those winter blues can be helped greatly by daily outdoor physical activity and increasing the amount of light in the home and working environments:

- Get as much daylight as possible through windows - try trimming bushes that are in front of windows, paint walls with light, bright colours, install brighter light bulbs, etc.
- Try to sit for periods of time at work or at home in front of sunlit windows. Maybe rearrange your workspace to be near a window - or make sure the lighting is good in your work area.
- Exercise daily, preferably outdoors - for example, a daily 20-minute walk around the block at lunchtime. If indoors, exercise in brightly lit environments.
- Try to stay on a regular sleep/wake cycle.
- If you are able, enjoy a winter holiday in a warm, sunny climate - but take care and use a good sunscreen!

Regular exercise is a great way to helps keep away those winter blues, whether outdoors or indoors. The gyms know that attendance will increase during the dark, winter months and now tend to offer a wide range of courses and activities.
So, keep active – and don't be a SAD victim!

Beating the Winter Blues
As the cold weather and dark nights creep in, motivation is harder to find and it's easy to let those fitness regimes slip.

There are many reasons to stay active over the winter months. Regular activity raises serotonin levels, helping to reduce common feelings of depression associated with the darker months. Also, research shows that you'll have less chance of catching the winter lurgies! One study suggests that exercising regularly and moderately can halve your risk of sore throats and those pesky winter colds.
Boost your motivation using these top tips for keeping workouts fresh and interesting over the winter:

Increase duration/intensity of exercise - add an extra few minutes to your routine or introduce short bursts of high intensity into your normal workout.

Adapt your regime to prevent fitness plateaus - the body quickly adapts to regular exercise, meaning you need to ring the changes to keep workouts challenging. Try new activities or changing speed and intensity in your existing routine.

Find yourself a workout buddy - the right partner can help you alleviate boredom and stick to your exercise regime. A partner can also motivate and challenge you to succeed.

Set realistic goals - choose a training goal appropriate to your fitness and skill level. Challenge yourself but be realistic about progress. Signing up for a race or other charity fitness event can give you the motivation needed to keep up your training.

Stay positive - a positive mental attitude can work wonders. Endorphin levels drop after just a couple of days of inactivity, reducing mood and energy, making you feel less inclined to exercise. Try to focus on the positive feeling you get after a good workout.

Exercise and Blood Pressure

Hypertension, or high blood pressure, is something that affects huge numbers of people. In the USA & UK around 20% of the population have hypertension – and around a quarter of those don't know they have it! High blood pressure doesn't give any warning signs and for this reason it is known as the 'silent killer'. Because there are often no symptoms, the only sure way you can know if your have hypertension is by having your blood pressure checked. Many people think they will feel dizzy, have headaches, suffer cramp in the legs, have a puffy face or red nose or just feel irritable when they have high blood pressure. Unfortunately, unless it is extremely high, none of these things happen – and many thousands of us are walking around with high blood pressure feeling fit and healthy. Very sadly, a stroke or heart attack is the first thing they know about it.

Blood pressure (BP) is complicated to put it mildly and trying to work what can make it go wrong still puzzles medical scientists. Think of a central heating system. Water is pumped through pipes to radiators all over the house. In the human body, the pump is your heart, the pipes are your arteries and veins, the radiators are your liver, kidneys, intestines, brain, skeleton, hands and feet. The central heating pump has to work hard to push water around the house. Likewise your heart has to work hard to push blood around your body. The amount of "push" the heart has to give with every beat is your *blood pressure*.

Just as the water pump has to work harder if your pipes and radiators get furred up, so it is with your heart if there is resistance to blood flowing through your arteries, veins and organs. This results in an increase in your BP and might be caused by stress, smoking, being overweight, drinking too much alcohol, eating too much salt and lack of exercise. Family history and taking the contraceptive pill are also factors known to be associated with elevated blood pressure.

The UK Coronary Prevention Group suggests that every adult over 25 years should have BP checked at least once every 5 years. Generally, women have their BP checked more often than this during routine visits to the doctor. However, far fewer men have regular BP checks.

The instrument used to check blood pressure is just an inflatable cuff with a gauge attached to it. The cuff is wrapped around your upper arm and pumped up in order to stop the flow of blood into your lower arm. The pressure cuff is slowly released and doctor or nurse will listen through a stethoscope, placed on your brachial artery near your elbow, for the sound of blood flow returning. When the first sound is heard this is the highest pressure (called 'systolic' BP) and is normally around 110-140mmsHg (the units are 'millimetres of mercury'). This then is the pressure of blood being pumped by the heart into your arteries. The last point where the sound is heard is the lowest pressure (called 'diastolic' BP) and is normally around 60-90mmsHg. This gives a good indication of the elasticity of your arteries and the resistance to blood flow.

So, if you have a BP of 120/80, the 120 is the highest pressure, when the heart contracts and the 80 is the lowest pressure between the heartbeats.

If your BP is below 140/90 this is usually considered normal. If it is over 160/100 this is generally considered too high and may need medical treatment. However, there is really no hard and fast rule because there is no definite point between high and low. Your doctor must decide what is best for you. For example, many doctors wouldn't treat a BP of 160/100 in a 75-year old, but likely would for a 35-year old.

Sometimes, blood pressure can be too low (less than 100/60). This is termed hypotension. Low BP is often accompanied by dizziness, lightheadedness or proneness to fainting when moving from lying or sitting to a standing position, particularly in a hot environment (e.g. sauna) or when emerging from a swimming pool. Whilst it is more common in elderly individuals low BP can occur in younger people. Both high and low blood pressure should always be checked out with your GP who will interpret the readings for any clinical significance.

The Exercise-Health-BP Connection

A brisk walk, cycle or swim will cause your systolic BP to rise from a resting level of around 120 to 150 or even 200. The harder you exercise, the higher it goes. Interestingly your diastolic BP remains roughly the same at rest as in exercise (around 80-90). But after exercise blood pressure falls – often below normal levels - and this effect can last up to several hours. Over time, regular exercise will help 'loosen up' your blood vessels thereby lowering your resting BP - rather like widening a water pipe lowers water pressure. This is one reason why you feel relaxed after physical activity.

Resistance training doesn't appear to be as effective as aerobic training in helping control blood pressure – and moderate aerobic exercise appears better than higher-intensity strenuous exercise. Many studies have shown that regular moderate exercise can help both prevent high blood pressure and help to cure it. In people with hypertension, research shows that moderate aerobic exercise can have a highly beneficial effect – and this can take place within the first few weeks. However, those with severe hypertension should first consult with their doctor before embarking on an exercise programme.

Also, when a person stops taking exercise, BP will return to its initial level. In other words, the BP-lowering effect of exercise depends on a regular (3 to 5 times a week) schedule of moderate physical activity

So, to help keep your blood pressure normal, watch your weight, cut down on alcohol and salt – and keep active!

The Stress–Exercise–Health Connection

Stress has been defined as "the rate of wear and tear in the body". The pace of modern-day living means that many of us lead stressful lifestyles. Whilst not all stress is harmful – indeed we need some degree of stress to stay alert and healthy – the sheer pace and pressures of life can, for many, become intolerable and have a serious effect on mental and physical wellbeing.

Our physiological 'fight or flight' responses that were essential for the survival of our primitive ancestors can be unhealthy in modern-day society. Stress and tension have been associated with heart disease, cancer, strokes, infection, asthma attacks, back pain, chronic fatigue, stomach & bowel disorders, headaches, insomnia, immune system depression (leading to more coughs, colds, flu & sore throats)... and the list is still being added to by medical scientists.

When something excites or threatens us, our brain activates the hormonal and nervous systems to handle the situation. The hypothalamus tells the anterior pituitary gland to secrete the hormone ACTH (adrenocorticotropic hormone) which travels to the adrenal gland and orders the release of other hormones called glucocorticoids (e.g. cortisol). These hormones are necessary for the body's response to stressful situations.

The nervous system activates the release of adrenaline (epinephrine) from the adrenal glands, which mobilise energy stores and increase heart rate and blood pressure. We are ready for action! However, if we have no physical outlet, these natural stress responses can have a deleterious effect on our health. For example, adrenaline makes the blood clot faster, an advantage in a fight but a disadvantage in the workplace or home where it can cause a heart attack. Glucose and fats are great energy sources when physical action is required but can damage and furr-up the arteries if they left in high quantities in the bloodstream in an up-tight sedentary person.

If you are a 'hot reactor' - the sort of person who easily flares up - then this stress response can often be exaggerated. Stress hormones flood out, heart rate and blood pressure soar, glucose and fats pour into the bloodstream and the blood clotting mechanisms are accelerated. If the 'hot reactor' is forced to regularly stew in their own juices, this sets the scene for major health problems. Prolonged exposure to stress hormones eventually suppresses the immune system and reduces our resistance to illness.

Around 50 years ago a psychologist called Dr Hans Selye, who pioneered the concept of stress, conducted a fascinating experiment to show the anti-stress benefits of exercise. He subjected 10 rats to a 4-week programme of mild electric shocks, flashing lights and loud noises. At the end of the month all the rats had died due to the stress that this had on their health. He then repeated the experiment and had 10 rats walk on a treadmill until they were in good physical condition, then subjected them to the same stressful programme. At the end of the month, all the rats were alive with no serious affects to their health. Dr Selye concluded that physical fitness helped to 'buffer' the health-destroying effects of stress.

Rather more recently a group of 36 physically inactive women were randomly assigned into either a walking or sedentary control group. The walking group exercised at a brisk pace for 45 minutes a day, 5 days a week for 15 weeks. After 6 weeks the walkers not only improved their heart-lung fitness but also improved their psychological wellbeing scores from an average of 70 (indicating a stress problem) to 81 (positive wellbeing) which was maintained throughout the 15-week study. The sedentary controls remained unchanged at around 70. A study of elderly women (average age 73 years) showed psychological wellbeing scores to be significantly higher amongst those who were regular walkers compared to those who were sedentary.

Regular moderate exercise has been consistently shown to minimise the effects of stress. It is relaxing, counters the tendency to form blood clots, uses the blood fats for energy, lowers stress hormone levels, reduces muscle tension and helps blood circulate more freely around the body. Studies have shown that a brisk walk is as effective in reducing stress and tension as a tranquilliser – and more long-lasting.

In general, moderate aerobic physical activity (e.g. walking, cycling, and swimming) seems to be more effective than vigorous, exhaustive activity or resistance exercise in helping reduce stress and tension.

Regular exercise favourably influences the hormones and neurotransmitters associated with depression and feelings of anxiety. Many researchers believe that the feeling of wellbeing that comes during and after exercise is due to mood-altering substances such as serotonin, dopamine, enkephalins and endorphins. There has been a special interest recently in endorphins, a morphine-like compounds released in the brain which can reduce pain, help normalise blood pressure and may induce a feeling of euphoria and wellbeing. It takes around 20 minutes for these endorphins to have an effect, hence the recommendation to take exercise for at least 20-30 minutes on a regular basis.

There's no doubt that regular exercise makes us feel better and better able to cope with the stresses and strains of daily life. A brisk 20-minute lunchtime walk can work wonders after a stressful morning.

Don't Get Bone Idle

Questions........
Do you take little or no exercise?
Do you smoke?
Do you drink a lot of alcohol?
Does your diet contain little or no calcium?
Do you have a fair skin and fine bone structure?
Do you have a family history of broken bones?
Are you a postmenopausal woman?
Are you taking excessive thyroid medication or high doses of cortisone-type drugs for conditions such as asthma, arthritis, or cancer?

The more times you answer "yes", the greater your risk of developing a bone-thinning disease that causes debilitating fractures of the spine, hip and wrist. This disorder is called 'osteoporosis' and affects millions of people worldwide. In the UK alone there are an estimated 3 million people with osteoporosis. It mainly affects people in middle and later life and is around six times more common in women than it is in men.

Osteoporosis is a condition in which bones are thinner than they should be - and thin bones are more likely to break. Gradual loss of calcium from bones is a normal process in middle and later life but if the loss is rapid or severe (as may happen to women at menopause) then the bones become brittle. They can break easily and are hard to heal. A fracture in a bone weakened by osteoporosis may require weeks, sometimes months, of hospitalisation. Some breaks never really heal properly and impair the physical ability of those affected, preventing them from leading a normal active life.

Our bony skeleton is basically a protein mix in which crystals of calcium and phosphates are embedded.
The majority of our bones consist of two parts: an outer shell-like layer of hard, compact bone (termed 'cortical' bone) and an inner region of sponge-like cancellous bone (termed 'trabecular' bone).
Cortical bone is very dense and provides a strong tubular structure with an outer fibrous covering called the 'periosteum', to which

ligaments, tendons and muscles are attached. Cortical bone accounts for around 80% of our total skeletal mass.

Trabecular bone is found mainly in the ends of the long bones of our arms and legs - which resemble the structure of an 'Aero' chocolate bar (see Diagram). This is a strong bony matrix, that gives lightness to our bones. Trabecular bone accounts for around 20% of our total bone mass.

The central shaft of long bones are basically hollow and contain the highly nutritious bone marrow, where, for example, most of our red blood cells are produced.

People with 'heavy frames' normally have higher levels of cortical bone than people with 'light frames'. The skeleton of males is on average around 30% heavier than females and about 10% higher in blacks than in whites.

From birth until death bone tissue is constantly being formed, broken down and re-formed in a process called 're-modelling'. The cells that build bones are called osteoblasts and those that break down bone and help create the bone shape are called osteoclasts.

During puberty, rapid bone growth occurs - our bones get longer, thicker and more dense. Our peak bone density occurs between the ages of 20 and 30. Once this has been achieved, the osteoclast and osteoblast activity remains in balance until around 45-50 years of age. After this, the osteoclast activity becomes greater than the osteoblasts and the person slowly begins to lose bone mass. A variety of genetic and lifestyle factors will slow or accelerate this process. For example, a woman going through the menopause will have accelerated loss of bone. The early occurrence of menopause by natural or surgical means also increases the risk of accelerated bone loss. This is because the protective effect of the female hormone oestrogen is lost since its natural production ceases after the menopause. Oestrogens act directly on bones, increasing their density. Studies have demonstrated that oestrogen replacement therapy can prevent the subsequent loss of bone by as much as 50%, whilst also helping alleviate menopausal symptoms. (Oestrogen may also reduce the risk of heart disease by as much as 50%; however there are some concerns that long-term use of oestrogen may increase the risk of breast cancer). Other menstrual problems, such as those caused by bulimia & anorexia, or excessive exercise, may also lead to loss of bone mass.

Prevention - the good news is that in the majority of cases osteoporosis is preventable - regular exercise and a healthy diet can make a great deal of difference to the health of our bones.

Regular Exercise promotes healthy bones - and helps prevent osteoporosis
It is well known that bone loss is much greater in those leading sedentary, inactive lifestyles. One study showed that when healthy individuals underwent complete bed rest for 10 weeks, they lost 10% of their bone mass!
Exercise, particularly weight-bearing and resistance exercise, which places a healthy stress on the bones is vital for maintenance of our total bone mass.
Weight-bearing activities such as walking, running and racket sports seem more effective than non-weight-bearing activities, such as cycling and swimming. Resistance exercises, such as lifting, carrying, pulling and pushing, or a gym programme designed to increase overall strength and muscle tone, will also have a highly beneficial effect on your bones, making them stronger and sturdier.
Encouraging children to play a variety of games and sports and lead active lifestyles, helps them to increase their peak bone mass, thus creating stronger and healthier bones. This stands them in good stead and helps reduce the risk of osteoporosis as they become older.
Regular exercise in later life is vital for healthy bones. As people age, they tend to become less physically active, which leads to a reduction in bone density and to the increased risk of fractures.

So, for good bone health make sure that:
- your diet contains adequate amounts of calcium from foods such as low-fat dairy foods, leafy vegetables, nuts and seeds
- don't smoke
- drink alcohol only in moderation
- don't become bone idle - take regular exercise!

Are You Fit to Sit?

Many of us spend several hours of every day sat down... at a desk, a table, a VDU, in a car, a train, a bus... or just flaked out in an armchair at the end of a tiring day - even when for most of it you've been sat down!

It's amazing how exhausting sitting all day can be!

Being sat down for several hours at a time causes a whole series of physiological changes to occur within your body. For example...

- your *muscles* will stiffen and ache.
- there's strain on your *neck, shoulders & back*, causing aches & pains. Your spine will change its curvature - from an upright and correct S-shape at the beginning of the day to a tilted-forward C-shape as you tire, putting added stress on your body.
- your *joints* stiffen...the liquid that lubricates them, called 'synovial fluid', is only produced through movement, so sitting all day causes your joints to 'dry out'. You'll notice this when you stand up after a long period sat down. Your body creaks and groans to begin with but as you loosen up with some stretching and mobilising movements the stiffness disappears as your joints become lubricated.
- your *blood circulation* becomes sluggish, with blood pooling in your lower limbs...this may cause your legs and feet to swell, causing aches and pains. It also puts strain on your heart, as it tries to pump the blood around the body. The mechanisms that return the blood from your extremities don't work so well when you're sat down for long periods - your breathing becomes shallow and your leg muscles are not helping to squeeze blood back through the veins to your heart. You may even feel faint, or light-headed when you stand up after a long period of sitting.
- this blood pooling in your lower limbs can also affect the *oxygen supply to your brain*, affecting concentration and mental alertness.

In short, a long day of sitting can leave you exhausted - and the last thing you feel like doing when you get home is an exercise workout! But really, that's exactly what your body needs to re-vitalise it.

Even better, if your lifestyle demands that you sit down for most of the day, then try to remember that your body needs a regular break in order to prevent these changes from occurring. A simple exercise programme of stretching and muscle toning, performed at regular intervals through the day, will help keep you alert, efficient and refreshed. Some of these exercises can even be done whilst you're sat down.

'Fit to Sit' Exercises

The following series of exercises can be done in your workplace or at home - you don't need to change into sportsgear. They will help prevent some of the problems caused by 'sitting down' all day, help relieve stress and keep you mentally alert, helping you to work more effectively and more efficiently. Throughout this programme, try to maintain good respiratory control by breathing in through the nose and out through the mouth in a deep but relaxed manner.

1. Stand n'Stretch
From a seated position with hands on knees, stand upright and stretch both arms above your head, breathing in as you do so. Hold this stretched position for 2-3 seconds, then slowly breathe out and return to sitting. Repeat 10 times.

2. Leg Swings
Stand sideways, hold on to back of chair with one hand for support. Keeping in an upright position:
Swing your outside leg *forwards and backwards* 10 times in a relaxed manner. Repeat with other leg. Do not bend forwards or swing upper body. This movement can be advanced by bringing the knee *upwards* towards the chest on the forward swing.

3. Heel-Toe Lifts
Standing with feet shoulder-width apart, hands by side, lift heels as far as possible, then rock back on to heels and lift front of foot as high as possible. Use chair-back for support. Repeat in a slow and controlled manner 10 times. (You can also do this exercise whilst you're sat down)

4. March-on-the Spot
At an easy pace, march on the spot, raising your knees as high as comfortably possible. Repeat for 20 steps.

5. Shoulder Shrugs
Sitting or Standing with feet shoulder-width apart: hands by side, slowly pull shoulders up towards ears as hard as possible, then push down as far as possible. Repeat 10 times.

6. Arm Circling
Standing with feet shoulder-width apart, arms outstretched sideways, slowly rotate arms backwards, downwards, forwards and upwards in a large circular manner. Repeat 5 times. Change direction and repeat a further 5 times.

7. Neck Rotation
Sitting or Standing with feet shoulder-width apart: hands by side, turn head slowly sideways to the right as far as comfortably possible, nod twice, and then turn head to the left and nod twice. Repeat 5 times.

8. Arm Raises
Sitting or Standing with feet shoulder-width apart: interlock fingers, turn palms outwards. Slowly raise hands above head without bending arms and stretch upwards .. breathing in. Hold for 3 seconds then lower .. breathing out. Repeat 5 times.

9. Chair Sit-Ups
From a normal seated position in your office chair, slither down so that you are sat near the front of the seat, reclining backwards, knees bent at 90° with feet flat on floor, hands on thighs. Now tighten your stomach muscles, curl forwards and slide your hands up your thighs to touch your knees. Briefly hold this 'half sit-up' position for 2 to 3 seconds, feeling the tension in your abdominal muscles, then return to relaxed recline. Repeat *up to* 10 times.

10. Wall Press
Stand facing wall, arm length away, feet shoulder width apart. Rest hands against wall and slowly bend elbows until nose touches wall. Slowly straighten arms and return to standing. Repeat *up to* 10 times.

Guidelines

Intensity: *don't work your muscles to exhaustion, exercise at a moderate level of exertion.* The exercises are not intended to make you hot and sweaty, but rather to stretch, loosen and tone your body so that you feel better and are ready return to the 'sedentary' job in hand. At no time should any pain or discomfort be felt in any part of your body. If any of the repetitions stated are too hard for you, then complete the exercise to a comfortable level of exertion *for you*.

Regularity: the exercise programme should be done as a whole, or in part, every day....in-between meetings..during your break..at regular slots during your working day...at home. For some, who may be sat at work for 8 hours a day, they are best performed 2, 3 or even more times a day.

Mix n'Match: either complete all the exercises at one go, or if you prefer, select 4 or 5 at a time to perform.

If your lifestyle is one of long periods of continuous sitting, this can lead to a whole series of adaptations to your body that are not good for your health and wellbeing......

So, in summary, make sure that you're fit to sit all day - and can handle the daily stresses and strains of sedentary living with vigour and alertness. Energy breeds energy!

How old do you feel..?

If you didn't know how old you are... how old would you think you are?

Your age tells us little about your health, wellbeing, appearance, energy levels or your physical fitness. As the saying goes: "You're as old as you feel".

Some people look and act much older than they are *all the time* - they seem to have aged prematurely! But others look remarkable, exude energy and exuberance - and look at least 10 years younger than they actually are.

Life expectancy figures have changed dramatically during this century.
In 1900 less than half the population lived to 65 whilst today around 80% live beyond 65 and over 50% live to see their 80th birthday. In fact by the year 2000, it's predicted that the fastest growing section of the population will be the *over-85s*.

However, although these trends are generally welcomed, there is great concern about the growing numbers of elderly people whose quality of life is severely affected by chronic illness and disease. Indeed, the US National Centre for Health Statistics estimates that 20% of the average American's life is spent in an 'unhealthy' state affected by disabilities, injuries and/or disease. That's over 15 years of illness! And for the majority of us most of that occurs in our later years. For example, amongst the over-65s - around 50% suffer from arthritis, 30% have high blood pressure, 26% suffer heart disease and 25% have problems with bones and joints. But it's worth remembering that many of these problems may start much earlier in life.
Whilst some illnesses, accidents and injuries strike without warning, it is now well established that *leading a healthy lifestyle can have a major influence on both our life expectancy and our quality of life as we get older.*

One famous US study, conducted on over 6,000 people in San Francisco showed a dramatic difference in disabling illnesses and death rate between those who followed SEVEN simple health habits and those who did not.

The health habits associated with both longevity and quality of life were:

1. **Not smoking** - smoking is without doubt dangerous to your health. If you don't smoke, don't start. If you do smoke, try your very best to stop.

2. **Regular exercise** -it's a staggering fact that you can reduce your risk of a heart attack by almost 50% by taking regular exercise - walking, gardening, swimming, dancing, golf, bowls, cycling, keep fit, etc. Regular aerobic activity supplemented by resistance exercises retains or restores mobility and the capacity for a free and independent life well into advancing years. In fact *those who age successfully invariably engage in daily routines that require physical activity.*

3. **Weight control** - when weight is more than 20% above or more than 10% below desirable, then health status declines. Keeping your weight in check is an invaluable way of staying healthy as time goes by.

4. **Moderate alcohol consumption** - whilst poor health is associated with heavy alcohol consumption, research shows that those who drink in moderation have lower levels of certain disease, such as heart disease. However, this should not be construed as a broad endorsement of drinking alcohol, since even moderate levels may lead to liver disease in the longer term. The best advice is to drink moderately or not at all - and don't save the weekends for a binge!

5. **A good daily breakfast** - in the California study, those who regularly ate a good breakfast - rather than just a cup of coffee or tea - experienced better health. Breakfast normally comes around 12 hours after the last (evening) meal when the body is in need of an energy boost.

6. **Regular meals** - the study showed that erratic eaters and 'snackers' had poorer health than those who had regular meals. The regular meal-eaters tended to eat more healthy wholesome

foods, whilst the 'snackers' were junk food eaters high in simple sugar & saturated fats and low in nutrients.

7. **Adequate sleep** - those who slept 7-8 hours per night were generally healthier than those who slept 6 hours or less (or, interestingly those who slept 9 hours or more per night!). Sleep is characterised by a series of alternating stages of rapid eye movement (REM) and quiet. The REM stage is often accompanied by dreams and by changes in heart rate, blood pressure and muscle tone. It accounts for around 20% of the night's total and if it is interrupted we get anxious and irritable. The deeper and quieter periods provide the rest necessary to recover from fatigue. The body seems to be able to handle missing the occasional night's sleep but if sleep is disturbed on several nights, the REM sleep stage is increased leading to restless and uncomfortable nights. Moderate exercise helps the body fall into deep sleep without altering the REM pattern. However, too much exercise can adversely affect our sleep patterns.

The Californian study showed that following just SIX of these habits we can add 10 YEARS to our lives. What's more those following all seven health habits were found to suffer HALF the rates of illness, injury and disability compared to those who did not practice any of them. Leading a healthy lifestyle can not only add years to your life but can greatly increase your quality of life in later years.

However, this information is not just aimed at people in their retirement years - it's aimed at ALL of us. Leading a healthy and active lifestyle will help ensure that we give ourselves the best chance possible of good health and fitness in the future.

Why do we gain weight when we age?

It's a well-known fact that as we get older, most of us put on weight. It is only the few who move into middle age can comfortably get into dresses and trousers we wore in our 20s. In fact across the UK population, on average there is a gradual increase in body weight of 3–5 kg (7-12lbs) *per decade* between the ages of 30 and 50 – the dreaded middle-age spread!

Why is this?
A major factor is that for most of us, after the age of 30 our general level of physiological function begins to slow down. We become less active and our aerobic fitness level decreases by around 5% per decade. Reactions slow, lung efficiency decreases, heart and circulation become less efficient, muscles lose strength (we actually lose muscle fibres (sarcopenia) as we age. On average we lose around 40-50% of our muscle mass between 30 and 65 years of age with a similar loss of bone mass. Since muscle (lean tissue) is a key calorie burner, our metabolism slows by as much as 5-10% per decade after 30. Not surprisingly therefore, if our eating habits remain the same, we become fat *storers* rather than fat *burners* – and we put on weight. Unfortunately, there is not an age-related decline in appetite!
But look at the graph below which demonstrates the remarkable effects of keeping fit and physically active. Even from early childhood there is a marked difference in general physiological function between sedentary and active individuals. During the *optimal timeslot* in our 20s, there is a 20-25% difference in the way our bodies work – and this extends well into our older years. In fact an active 65 year-old can have the physiology of a person more than 20 years younger!
Staying fit and active maintains muscle mass which helps prevent the lowering of metabolic rate, which in turn helps prevent the age-related weight loss so commonly seen in our society.

Whilst the most common method of weight loss is dieting, the long-term success rate of this method is quite poor. Only about 10-20% of those who lose weight by reducing calories maintain their full weight loss over the longer term Taking exercise is strongly associated with better long-term weight control than dieting alone.

A study recently published in the International Journal of Obesity surveyed of over 5,000 middle-aged men and women compared improvements in aerobic fitness – measured by the time walked on a treadmill with the gradient increasing every minute - with changes in body weight over an 8-year period. Even those who only marginally improved their aerobic fitness level (i.e. a one-minute improvement in treadmill time) gained on average only 0.6 kilograms (1.3lbs) compared to those who showed no improvement in fitness who gained on average almost 5kgs (11lbs) over the 8 years.

Each one-minute improvement in treadmill time reduced the chance of a 6kg (1stone) weight gain by 15% in men and by 10% in women and the chance of a 10kg (3 stones) gain by 21 percent in both men and women.

It should be noted, however, that *improvements* in fitness level were necessary to minimize weight gain; simply maintaining a given fitness level was not sufficient to ward off the slow increase in body weight through middle age. Indeed, these and other recent findings suggest that increasing amounts of physical activity may be necessary to effectively maintain a constant body weight with increasing age.

Thus, it seems that increased physical activity and fitness play more of a role in minimizing age-related weight gain and preventing significant weight gain than in promoting weight loss. Many of the chronic and disabling diseases now prevalent in our society may be in part attributed to an increase in age-related weight gain.

The message is clear. For long-term weight control, regular exercise is a must.

Regular Exercise Promotes Healthy Ageing

Britain is ageing at an unprecedented rate. In 1900, less than 5% of the population were over 65 years of age but now that figure is approaching 20%. It is estimated that by 2020, 25% of the nation will be over-65. The statistics are even more remarkable for the oldest group of people, namely those over 85, who are the most rapidly growing section of our society. We have been warned by experts on many occasions about the increasing costs of providing health and social care for the elderly.

However, it's not all bad news. Recent research shows that a healthy lifestyle can have a major impact on the ageing process. Ageing does not have to be something negative that happens when we get older. In fact we can do much to influence how our bodies age and one of the most powerful lifestyle interventions is regular physical activity. Indeed, a recent World Health Organisation Report concluded that physical activity is the single most effective means for individuals to positively influence their own health and functional abilities and thus maintain a high quality of life in old age.

So, what might some of these benefits be? Well, for example, even a single bout of exercise, such as a brisk walk or swim can improve sleep, help lower blood pressure and regulate blood glucose levels. Regular participation improves cardiovascular functioning, increases muscle strength and enhances balance and flexibility. The physiological benefits of exercise apply equally to men and women of all ages. In addition, there are significant psychological benefits for elderly persons. The feeling of having more energy and vitality, being better able to relax and having not only more self-confidence but also more 'body-confidence' are key factors. The social benefits of joining a walking group, a swimming club or one of the many other senior citizen organisations that promote healthy lifestyles provide wonderful opportunities for seniors to widen their social networks, form new friendships and acquire new positive roles during their retirement.

However, although the benefits of exercise for the elderly are well established, it is reported than a huge percentage of our population over 50 takes very little leisure-time exercise at all! Indeed, the number of inactive older adults increases as age increases and in some groups, especially older women, the percentage may be as high as 60-70%!

So why? What's the problem?
One of the main reasons is that *reliable* information about these health benefits has yet to reach many older people. The messages are often muddled, and there are too many myths and misconceptions, such as:

Myth 1: I'm too old to start exercising
Many people really believe this. However, exercise has been shown to benefits people of all ages, including those in their 90s and even 100s!

Myth 2: You have to be healthy to exercise
Becoming more physically active will improve quality of life for the vast majority of older people. Indeed, it may be most effective in people with chronic conditions and diseases. In our own laboratories here in Chester we are undertaking research, together with surgeons from the local hospital, on elderly patients suffering from a disabling condition affecting the lower limbs called peripheral artery disease. Most patients were unable to walk more than a couple of minutes on our treadmill at a very slow speed before having to stop with chronic leg pains. They were all on a waiting list for surgery. However, after 3 months of a gently progressive walking programme, together with changes in smoking and eating habits where appropriate, the results were startling. One 75-yr old lady who walked for less than ONE minute initially, was able to walk for a full THIRTY minutes at a fairly brisk pace – what's more, she was taken off the waiting list. So, how's that for improvement in quality of life – she was a totally different person – full of life and full of confidence!

Myth 3: You have to be fit to exercise
Perhaps surprisingly, many elderly people feel that they are not fit enough to join an exercise class. One common misconception is that those who go to such classes are fit - and that they would be embarrassed. In fact, classes such as Rosemary's are tailor-made for unfit elderly people and they would be with others similarly out-

of-shape. Those individuals would get expert advice on how to improve their fitness gradually and effectively.

Myth 4: You need special clothing and equipment:
Safe and effective exercise can be performed in loose-fitting everyday clothes and comfortable shoes. Even strength training can be done at home with inexpensive equipment, with household items or just using your body weight.

Myth 5: no pain, no gain
Many older adults learned about exercise when it was believed that it had to hurt to be of any benefit. We now know better – and if it hurts, you're probably doing too much of the wrong type of exercise.

Keeping on the move with a wide variety of physical activities is a great way for elderly people to stay in shape. If you have elderly relatives – pass on the message: *'regular exercise promotes healthy ageing'*.

Music Boosts Exercise Performance

We all recognise that music can have a huge effect on our mood and emotions. We are all aware that different types of music will have totally different effects on our bodies.

Music can help us relax, cope with anxiety, depression and tolerate pain (even labour pain). It can make us feel more energetic and enthusiastic, heighten our sense of pleasure - or it can make us feel sad. It can help us sleep better, think more clearly, study and work more effectively. The magic of music is a truly amazing.

So, it probably comes as no surprise to you that music can boost your exercise performance and make your workout a more positive experience – even when it hurts!

Many of us find that when we exercise, hearing our favourite tunes or listening to rhythmic beat music will encourage us to exercise that bit harder or go that little bit longer when we feel like giving up. Elite athletes have known this for many years and regularly use music when training as a strong motivator to perform all-out, exhaustive exercise. But also, they use different music to help them relax and stay calm before a big event.

But these days, it's not just for the athletes, exercising to music is a very effective way for enhancing the exercise experience for all of us – whether it be wearing a personal iPod/MP3 player headset in the gym or when out for a walk or run, or listening to loudspeaker music in group exercise classes.

Researchers at London's Brunel University studied the effects of exercising on a treadmill while listening to a selection of music, including songs by Queen, the Red Hot Chilli Peppers and Madonna. They were asked to keep in strict time with the beat. They showed that carefully selected music enhanced endurance performance by around 15 per cent and helped the participants derive greater pleasure from exercising, even when they were working out at a very high intensity. The researchers concluded that four factors contribute to the motivational qualities of a piece of music whilst exercising:

a) Rhythm - the tempo or speed of the music
b) Harmony and melody of the music
c) Cultural impact
d) Association with other feelings or events – e.g. Chariots of Fire is often associated with Olympic glory.

Music tends to have a steady tempo to it, often measured in "beats per minute". A simple observation is that most music is in the range of 50-200 beats per minute, which interestingly is roughly the same range of our heartbeats. Also, in general the tempo of a piece of music roughly equates with the heartbeat associated with the corresponding physical state or emotion which the music suggests.
Slow music (e.g. playing at less than 60 beats/min) is often very relaxing and introspective – but can also be very depressing! When the beat speeds up to 60-80 beats per minute this tends to relate to is a calm and relaxed mood, 80-100 is moderately alert and interested. 100 upwards is increasingly lively, excited or agitated and, 80-120 (quite a common tempo) relates to vigour and excitement whilst 120-160 is commonly associated with generates very lively and energetic moods. The faster the music beat, the harder we tend to exercise – to keep up with the rhythm. So in a typical aerobics workout, the heartbeat and music beat are often both around 130-160 beats per minute, whereas in a heavy, more exhaustive workout, both the tempo and heart rate are usually higher.

How does it work?

Basically there are three ways:
- Music can lower your perception of the physical effort you are making. It can trick your mind into feeling less tired during a workout and also encourage positive thoughts. So you feel less pain.
- Matching the music beat to the tempo of the exercise helps you move more rhythmically and even reduce the oxygen required by up to 6% - making you much more efficient in your movement – so you don't feel as tired.
- The rhythmical qualities of music can improve your technique and make you a more efficient exerciser – and make you feel more energetic.

Last year, there was even a London's Music Half-Marathon - the Sony Ericsson *Run to the Beat*. The music that was played during the run to the beat was scientifically selected to match the physiological and psychological demands of a half marathon event. Competitors generally reported substantial benefits from running to music – both mentally and physically.

How do you pick the music suitable for you when exercising?

Brunel University's Dr Kostas Karageorghis suggests the following:

- To find out the beats per minute of your favourite tracks put the title of the song and 'beats per minute' into an internet search engine and it will tell you. This will help you build your playlists
- Match the music to the activity you are undertaking and the psychological effect you want to experience. For example, loud, fast, rhythmical, percussive, bass-driven music is great for psyching yourself up before and during more strenuous interval training.
- Consider the tempo - is the speed of the music and its rhythm (pattern of beats over time) ideal for your running cadence?
- How intense is the activity: generally speaking you will need faster music if you are running at a faster pace (music of 130-150 bpm is ideal for high-intensities).
- Does the tempo of the music match your expected heart rate during your workout?
- Has the music got a rhythm (beat) that makes you want to exercise?
- Do the lyrics contain positive affirmations of running such as "keep on running", "born to run" or "run to the beat"? Other positive statements such as "moving on up" or "I believe" also lead to positive motivational consequences.
- Does the music create imagery in your mind that is motivational; maybe through associations the piece has within popular culture (e.g. the "Rocky" film series soundtrack) or through personal memories?
- Does the music remind you of your adolescence, early adulthood or another part of your life that stimulates positive feelings for you?

- Does the music possess a pleasing melody and harmony (combination of notes played at the same time that shapes the emotional "colour" of the music) which improves your mood? Generally speaking, major (happy) harmony is more appropriate for exercise than minor (sad) harmony.
- Does the music emanate from the genre (e.g., 'pop', 'rock', 'urban', or 'dance' etc.) which you grew up with and can identify with?
- Does the music make you feel excited or 'psyched-up'?
- Does the music evoke a positive state of mind?
- Does the music make you feel confident and does it promote motivational thoughts?
- Are you familiar with the music without finding it tiresome owing to overexposure to it?

Playing carefully selected your music that suits *you* can be of huge benefit to help you achieve your health and fitness goals.

Even if all it does is make your workout that bit more enjoyable, it's a simple, pain-free trick that can help you stick with your programme long-term ... and that means better health!

So, now create a great playlist that works for you!

Gain - without Pain!

Speaking to a group of international athletes a few months ago, one world-class triathlete and regular Iron-Woman competitor commented privately to me that she would train intensively on a daily basis to reach competitive levels – and judged herself to be at peak fitness when her periods had stopped! Asked if she felt that this might be detrimental to her health she shrugged: "Maybe – but it's the only way to win medals!"

The pressure to train hard and strive for ultra-slimness is not necessarily confined to top-level athletes. The plethora of fun runs and other charity events with the commitment to train hard in order to produce best performance may sometimes damage rather than enhance health. The intensive training regimes in many gyms where the 'no pain, no gain' philosophy still exists can significantly increase the risk of injury.

Those who engage in a programme of regular moderate exercise gain significant benefits to their health and wellbeing, have more energy and increased vitality. However, exercising too hard, too often, can be harmful to health. If you're overdoing it, this can cause you to pick up an array of minor illnesses such as coughs, colds, sore throats, cold sores and flu, be more prone to injury and for females there may be other complications, such as irregular periods and loss of bone density.

Research shows that females who are highly physically active, in particular those involved in sports that require a low body fat percentage for success, increase their chances of either a delayed onset of menstruation (menarche), irregular periods (oligomenorrhea) or complete cessation of periods (amenorrhea). For example, ballet dancers and gymnasts, who are normally very lean, report far more incidences of menstrual irregularities and a higher mean age for menarche compared to other girls. One recent study showed that around 40% of female athletes in endurance-type sports have some menstrual irregularity. Ballet dancers, gymnasts and female distance runners also report more eating disorders than normal, which worsens the problem.

When menstrual function is irregular or absent in premenopausal women, there is an increased risk of bone loss and of injury to joints, muscles, ligaments and tendons when participating in high-intensity exercise.

Some researchers also now believe that the body somehow 'senses' when the physical stresses are high and energy levels are inadequate to sustain a pregnancy, and thus cease ovulation in order to prevent conception.

This condition has been termed by exercise scientists as the 'Female Athlete Triad' and consists of amenorrhea, osteoporosis and disordered eating. Whilst it was originally identified as a problem associated with elite athletes, it is now becoming more common in girls and women who are overly committed to getting extremely fit and very thin. The condition often results as pressures are placed on young women to achieve or maintain unrealistically low body weight. This is something that can and should be avoided - if girls and women are made aware of the potential dangers and are able to recognise the early warning signs.

A recent UK survey reported that many athletes believed that disordered eating practices are harmless and that losing weight by any means will enhance performance! In reality, the reverse is true – that inadequate calorie intake and disordered eating practices impair physical performance and affect health. Problems result from a depletion of energy stores, dehydration, loss of muscle mass, low blood sugar levels, electrolyte abnormalities, anaemia, amenorrhea and osteoporosis. Also, the study reported that many female athletes did not regard amenorrhea as a problem – indeed several reported using it an indicator of an adequate training intensity!

However, it is known that the low concentrations of ovarian hormones in amenorrhea and oligomenorrhea are strongly associated with reduced bone mass and increased rates of bone loss. This loss of bone in young women is similar to bone loss in postmenopausal women and leads to osteoporosis.

As always, prevention is better than cure. And for those girls and women engaged in regular vigorous exercise at whatever level of ability and performance, knowing how to recognise the early warning signals of over-exercising and then taking informed action to make sure things get better – not worse - is an invaluable skill in promoting personal health, fitness and wellbeing.

The message is the same for those just beginning an exercise programme, keen to lose weight, who think that 'more is better' and go completely 'o.t.t.' and overdo it. So instead of feeling good after exercise, they feel absolutely shattered – and have difficulty getting out of bed the morning after! For example, most of us would have difficulty jogging for 30 minutes – and would likely suffer - but most of us could walk briskly for half an hour and get significant benefits. Over-enthusiasm at the gym can sometimes take days to recover from – a sensible workout is one that doesn't leave you totally exhausted – but rather with an after-glow that makes you feel good.
There are lots of examples of physical activities, such as gardening, cleaning the car, cleaning windows, general housework – and even ironing – which are great for improving overall mobility and fitness without overdoing it.

The key message is that exercise is great for health and wellbeing, and will help you tone up and slim down. But make sure that you exercise well within your capabilities – and don't overdo it. Remember, there is gain, without pain!

Laughter – a great form of exercise!

"A merry heart maketh good medicine"
(Proverbs)

Laughter is the physiological response to humour. To the scientist, laughter consists of two parts – a set of gestures and the production of a sound. When you laugh, your brain pressures you to conduct both these activities at the same time. When you laugh heartily, 15 facial muscles contract, including the *zygomatic* muscle in your upper lip (your 'smiling' muscle). Also, your breathing is upset by the epiglottis in your throat half-closing your larynx. Air intake then comes in spasms, making you gasp. In extreme laughter, the tear ducts are activated making you cry, so that while your mouth is opening and closing struggling for air, your face becomes moist and often red (or even purple!) The noises that accompany this bizarre behaviour range from sedate giggles to boisterous guffaws.

Laughter is a reflex, and reflexes evolved in our species because they have survival value. The body/mind is a single entity and the physical act of laughing informs the mind that all is well. It seems that we are hard-wired to laugh. Laughter is one of the keys to unlocking a free pharmacy that has virtually no negative side effects.

Laughter is healthy and its benefits are many:

- Laughter strengthens your immune system by increasing the number of natural killer cells, gamma-interferon (a disease-fighting protein), T-cells (a major part of your immune response) and B-cells (which make disease-destroying antibodies). All these cells have the power to destroy tumours and viruses. Laughter also increases the concentration of salivary immunoglobulins (Igs) which defend against infectious organisms entering through your respiratory tract. In simple terms laughter helps your immune system function more effectively making you more able to fight off diseases.

- Laughter is a great way to handle stress. Problems that can be laughed at can't so easily overwhelm you. At a biochemical level, laughter provides a safety valve that shuts off the supply of stress hormones - which if left unchecked in the bloodstream will suppress your immune system, increase the number of blood platelets (which can cause obstructions in your arteries) and raise your blood pressure.

- Laughter is the shortest distance between people. The right sort of laughter can dissolve the barriers of awkwardness and embarrassment that sometimes block communication. Laughter helps - whether talking 1-to-1 or in groups.

- Laughter leads to learning – smiles and laughter help keep you interested and motivated whether it's in an exercise class or in other situations. The adrenaline that accompanies laughter seems to help fix information in those little protein stacks of memory – so you remember those hints and tips more easily.

- Laughter is helpful to those coping with disaster situations. The tougher the job, often the blacker the humour. Firefighters, doctors, nurses, paramedics, and police often use black humour to lighten the impact of the horrors with which they are sometimes confronted.

- The Latin for laughter is *ridiculum*, and an ability to see the ridiculous in others and ourselves is a wonderful survival tool.

The American Association for Therapeutic Humour reckon that the psychological benefits of laughing are quite amazing. Pent-up emotions such as anger, hate, sadness, stress and fear can all be dissipated by laughter. Laughter is cathartic. That's why some people who are stressed out go to a funny movie or a comedy show, so they can laugh away the negative emotions. The brilliant movie 'Patch Adams', in which Robbie Williams portrayed a real-life 'funny-doc' showed to millions of us the impact that laughter can have and increasingly mental health professionals are recognising the importance of 'laughter therapy' – which teaches people how to laugh.

Laughter is great exercise. Researchers estimate that laughing 100 times is equal to 10 minutes on a rowing machine or 15 minutes on an exercise bike! Laughing can be a total body workout. It gives your diaphragm, abdominal, respiratory, facial, leg and back muscles a good workout. That's why you often feel exhausted after a long bout of laughing – you've just had an aerobic workout!

Heard the one about……..

Check your Fitness

Fitness is not merely a matter of working out or eating the right foods but rather the cumulative effect of our lifestyle. Most of us would like an idea of just how fit we are and answering a few simple questions and stepping onto and off the bottom step of a flight of stairs at home can help tell you.

1. How many times a week do you take moderately vigorous exercise for 20 minutes or more?
If the answer is less than 3, you're probably not at the top of your form. You need to work up a sweat at least 3 times a week to maintain a good level of health-related fitness

2. Are you physically active in your job?
If you spend much of your day moving around, walking, climbing stairs, lifting and carrying packages you're probably already in reasonable shape. A study on London bus drivers and conductors revealed that the sedentary drivers were more than twice as likely to have a heart attack than the conductors who were walking up and down stairs all day.

3. Do you watch your weight?
A little bit of surplus fat will not shorten your lifespan but if you are carrying several stones more than you should for your height and body build then this puts extra strain, not just on your heart but on all your body organs and joints. Two extra stones of fat will reduce your aerobic fitness by around 20%!

4. Have you had your BP checked recently?
Good fitness offers benefits for everyone but particularly for those who blood pressure is too high. When you have your BP checked you are given two readings (for example 130/85). The first is called systolic BP and indicates the pressure in your arteries when your heart pumps out blood. Ideally this should be around 110-140mmsHg. The second (or bottom) reading is termed diastolic BP and gives an indication of the elasticity of your arteries. Ideally this reading should be between 90-110mmsHg. If your BP is too high you should take steps to reduce it. Depending what causes the condition, you may be

able to reduce it by a combination of diet (e.g. reducing salt and saturated fat intake), moderate aerobic exercise and appropriate medication prescribed by your GP. In some instances, your doctor might even prescribe exercise alone!

5. Are you generally positive in your outlook?
Stress, depression and a negative outlook on life can lower your body's resistance to disease – and one of the best ways to alleviate stress and depression is aerobic exercise. The endorphin-release caused by exercise can really help lift your spirits.

6. Do you make time to relax every day?
People who can relax and switch-off suffer from fewer illnesses. Whether it's aerobic exercise or sport, working in the garden, strolling through the park or playing with the kids, we all need some 'play-time' to stay at the peak of our health. Exercise can really help you relax and give your body and mind some quality time.

7. Are you doing anything to control your cholesterol levels?
Cholesterol deposited in the arteries leads to heart disease – the No. 1 cause of death in the UK. And the UK is still one of the world leaders when it comes to heart disease – with more and more females suffering at an earlier age. Eating a healthy, low fat diet and taking regular aerobic exercise will not only lower cholesterol but will produce more HDLs in your blood (the 'good' cholesterol that helps prevent the arteries from furring up). So, if you need another reason to exercise scientists have discovered it makes cholesterol less dangerous.

8. When you workout, do workout flat-out?
The health benefits of exercise are from moderate bouts of exercise, not exhaustive workouts. If you're overdoing it you can literally wear down your body and lower your resistance to disease. So don't aim to hit maximum effort – take it easy and enjoy your exercise. The chart below gives you an idea of how hard to exercise.

Perceived Exertion Scale		Exercise & CHD:

Perceived Exertion Scale
6
7 Very, very light
8
9 Very light
10
11 Fairly light
12
13 Somewhat hard
14
15 Hard
16
17 Very hard
18
19 Very, very hard
20 Maximal

Exercise & CHD:
Risk v Benefit ⬇

LIGHT EXERCISE
Some CHD benefits
but minimal fitness improvement

⬇

MODERATE EXERCISE
Both CHD and fitness benefit
With minimal risk

⬇

INTENSE EXERCISE
For those who desire high fitness.
Can precipitate heart attack
in high risk
Individuals.

9. Can you take this 3-minute step test without getting overly tired or breathless?

The test is quite safe for anyone who is healthy and moderately active. If you have any medical problems or are unsure about trying this test, please consult your doctor before attempting the step test.

If you experience breathless or distress during the step test, please stop, sit down and recover.

Use the bottom step of a flight of stairs. Step on and off in an Up-2, Down-2 rhythm for exactly 3 minutes at a steady rate of 24 steps/min (i.e. 2 steps every 5 seconds) – so in 3 minutes you will have stepped onto and off the step a total of 72 times. After stopping, rest for 30 seconds, find your pulse and count the beats for another 30 seconds. Check out your score with the Table below.

	Age			
	20-29	30-39	40-49	50+
Males	**Beats/30secs**			
Excellent	34-36	35-38	37-39	37-40
Good	37-40	39-41	40-42	41-43

83

Average	41-42	42-43	43-44	44-45
Fair	43-47	44-47	45-49	46-49
Poor	48-59	48-59	50-60	50-62
Females				
Excellent	39-42	39-42	41-43	41-44
Good	43-44	43-45	44-45	45-47
Average	45-46	46-47	46-47	48-49
Fair	47-52	48-53	48-54	50-55
Poor	53-66	54-66	55-67	56-66

What to do next

Poor to Fair – you need to undertake an aerobic beginners exercise programme.

Average – you need to exercise more regularly – ideally 20mins/day, 3days/wk

Good – You're in good shape – but there's still room for improvement

Excellent – keep up the good work.